# DIABETIC RECIPES FOR ONE AND TWO

MICHELLE BERRIEDALE-JOHNSON

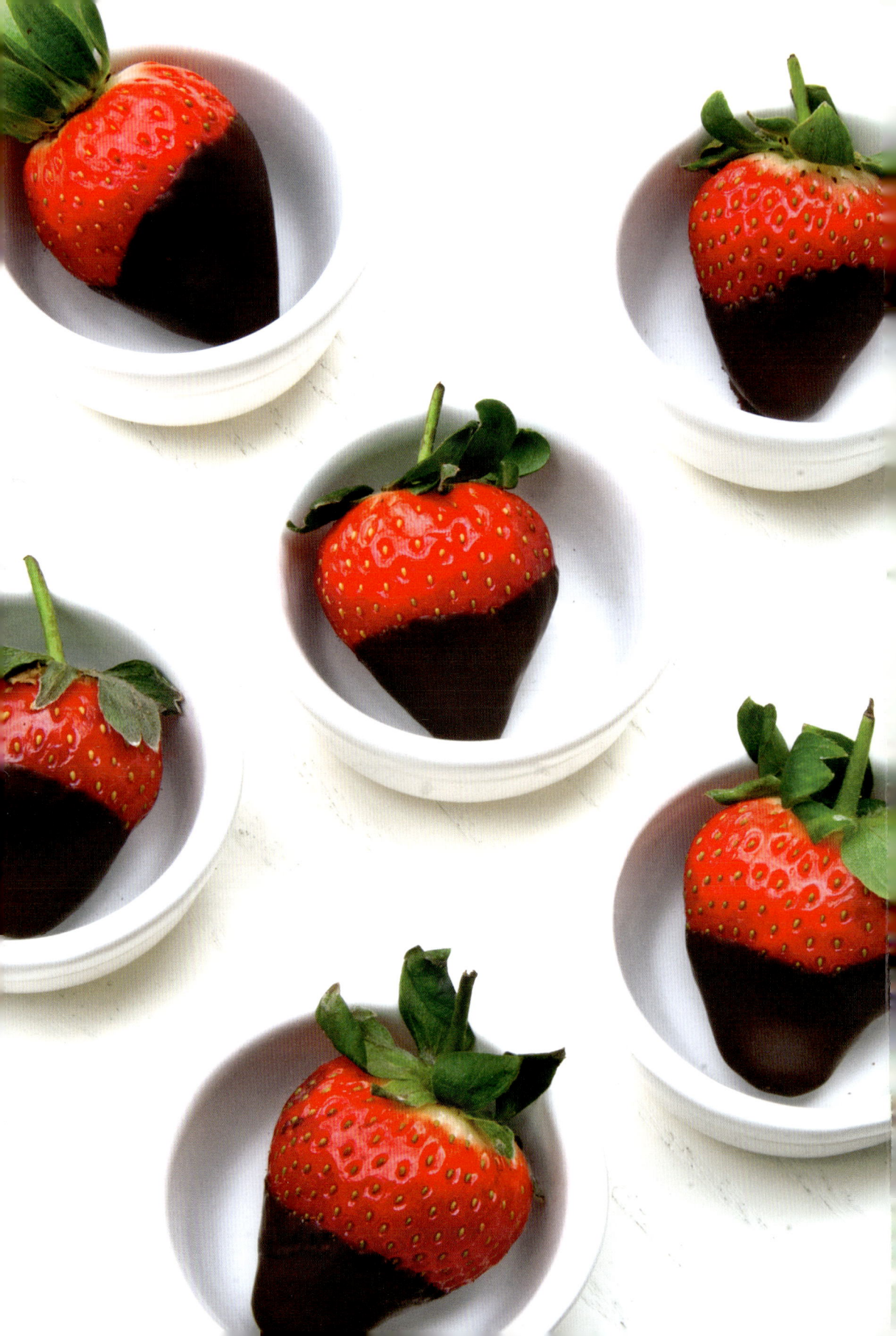

# DIABETIC RECIPES FOR ONE AND TWO

MICHELLE BERRIEDALE-JOHNSON

GRUB STREET • LONDON

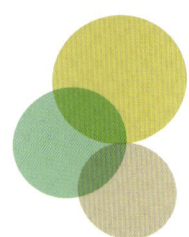

Published in 2023 by
Grub Street
4 Rainham Close
London SW11 6SS
www.grubstreet.co.uk
email: food@grubstreet.co.uk
Twitter: @grub_street

Text copyright © Michelle Berriedale-Johnson, 2013, 2023
Copyright this edition © Grub Street 2023
Published originally under the title *Diabetic Cooking for One and Two* in 2013

Cover design by Myriam Bell
Photography by Michelle Garrett
Food styling by Jayne Cross

The moral right of the author has been asserted

A CIP record for this title is available from the British Library

ISBN 978-1-911714-00-2

All rights reserved. No part of this publication may be reproduced, stored in a retrieval system, or transmitted in any form or by any means, electronic, mechanical, photocopying, recording or otherwise, without the prior permission of the copyright owner.

Printed and bound by Finidr, Czech Republic

# CONTENTS

Introduction   6
- What is Diabetes?   8
- Symptoms, diagnosis and medical treatment   8
- Alternative approaches   9
- Nutritional therapy   11
- Blood sugar control: hyper and hypoglycaemia   11
- Diet   12
- Glycaemic Index and Glycaemic Load   13
- The good, the bad and the ugly   14
- Alcohol   15
- Alternative sweeteners   15

Recipes
- Soups and Starters   17
- Eggs   31
- Pasta   39
- Seafood and Fish   47
- Beef   63
- Lamb   73
- Pork   83
- Poultry and Game   89
- Vegetables, Salads and Vegetarian Dishes   99
- Festive Meals   115
- Desserts   123
- Baking   137

Index   150

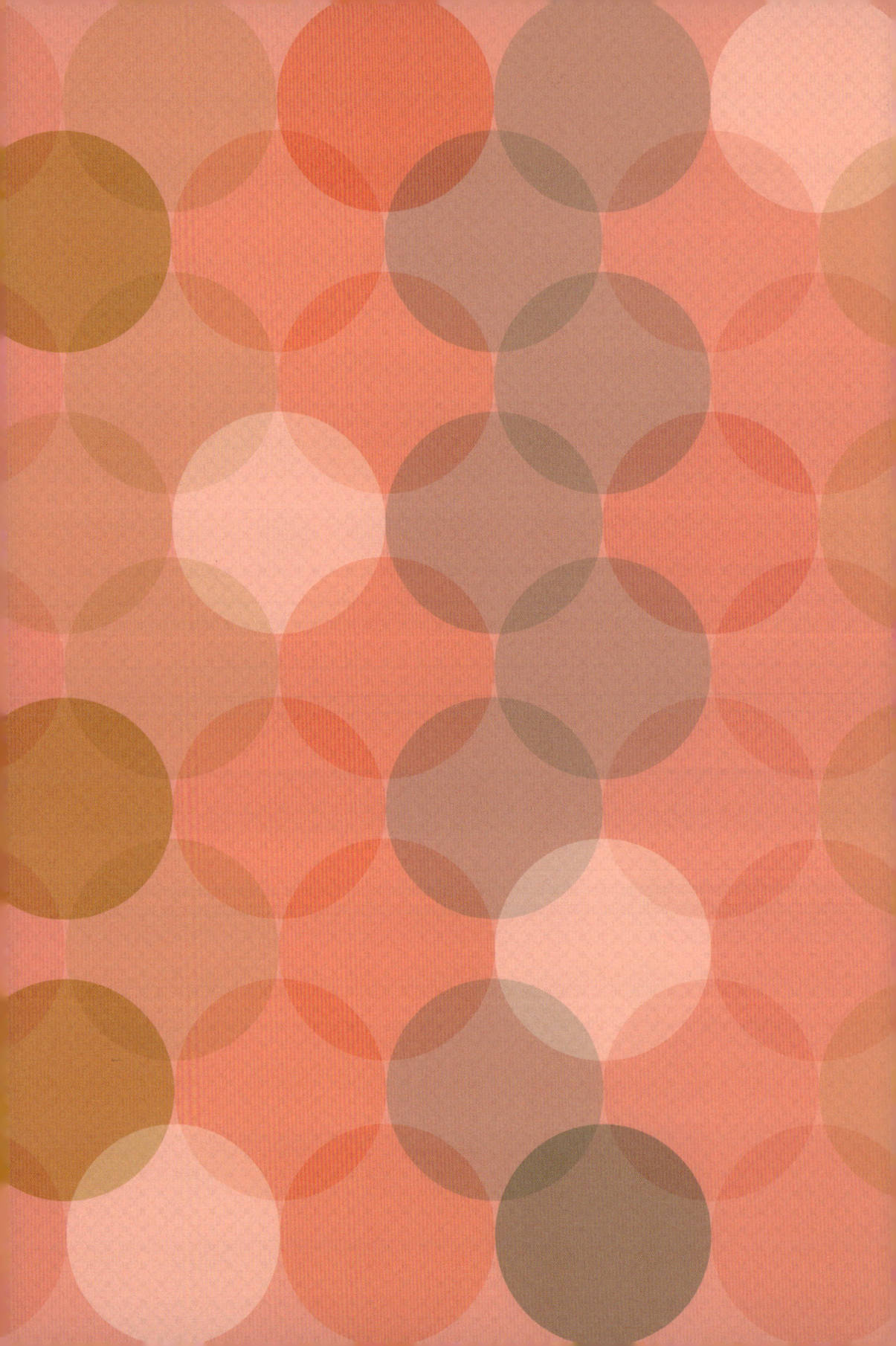

# INTRODUCTION

# INTRODUCTION

The chances are that if you have bought this book, you will have lived with diabetes for some time and so are pretty familiar with this condition. But just in case I will run through the basics.

## What is diabetes?

The name, *diabetes mellitus*, comes from the Greek for a 'siphon' and 'honey' because in diabetics, the glucose circulating in the bloodstream cannot be properly absorbed and therefore the urine tastes sweet.

Glucose (a simple form of sugar) is our body's main fuel; it provides both our muscles and our brains with the energy they need to function. We absorb glucose from the foods that we eat. These are initially broken down by enzymes in our saliva as we chew, and then further by our stomach acids and by the digestive juice from the pancreas and gall bladder in the gut. At this point glucose is absorbed through the gut wall into the blood stream and then moves on to the liver where it is converted into glycogen (the form of sugar which actually delivers the energy) and stored until needed.

However, the glucose cannot enter the cells in the liver without the help of insulin, a hormone that is manufactured in the pancreas and released in response to rising glucose levels in the blood. Once in the blood stream the insulin attaches to cells through 'insulin receptors' that precipitate chemical changes in the cell walls and allow the glucose to enter the cells and be converted into glycogen or energy – not unlike two space ships docking to allow the crew to transfer.

In non-diabetics, this process is automatic; in diabetics the process is impaired. In Insulin Dependent, or Type 1, Diabetics (IDDM) the pancreas fails to produce any insulin at all; in Non-insulin Dependent, or Type 2, Diabetics (NIDDM) the pancreas does not produce enough insulin to do the job properly.

There is now a third insulin-related condition that is becoming increasingly common, known as Insulin Resistance (also known as Metabolic Syndrome or Syndrome X) in which the pancreas does produce insulin but the insulin does not react properly with the cells to allow the transfer of sugar into the cells for conversion into glycogen/energy. As a result the levels of sugar in the blood continue to rise and the pancreas pumps out more and more insulin both of which continue to circulate in the blood affecting kidney function and causing weight gain and general un-wellness.

## Symptoms, diagnosis and medical treatment

In IDDM the failure of the pancreas to produce insulin is usually sudden and complete and occurs usually among children or those under the age of 30 and usually in people who are relatively slim.

Symptoms are fairly obvious and easily recognised:
- Intense thirst and the passing of unusually large amounts of urine. If the levels of glucose in the blood are too high the kidneys cannot filter it all so some escapes into the urine,

thickening the urine which then needs to draw extra water from the body's cells to allow it to pass. Thus extra urine is being passed so a dehydrated body needs to drink more.
- Constipation – an inevitable result of dehydration.
- Tiredness and weight loss. The body is not getting enough energy in the form of glucose so will break down other cells in an attempt to replace this energy source.
- Blurred vision. If the blood is thick and sugary it will have difficulty getting through the tiny capillaries in the eyes causing vision to become blurred.
- Pins and needles in the extremities. As with the eyes, thick sugary blood can affect nerve endings in the extremities.

A positive urine test (e.g. high in sugar) will be followed by a blood test (blood taken from the vein). Blood sugar should be below 7.8millimoles (mmol) per litre and should not rise above 11mmol/litre. If you fall within the criteria of age, size, symptoms and test results you will probably be put on insulin immediately and offered dietary advice.

NIDDM or Type 2 diabetes is more likely to occur in the middle aged or elderly especially if they are overweight, take little exercise and eat a lot of refined sugars and carbohydrates in their diet.

In NIDDM symptoms are very much less obvious and, indeed, you may have no symptoms at all. However, this does not mean that you can ignore NIDDM. Prolonged high blood sugars can lead to a significantly increased risk of heart attack and stroke, will eventually impair the function of any area of the body with small capillaries which get clogged up with sticky, sugary blood (the eyes, the kidneys and the extremities in particular), and will impact on every aspect of your health.

Therefore, if you are overweight, have a family history of diabetes, have high blood pressure or are suffering from a number of ill-defined health problems, it is well worth getting your blood sugar levels checked.

There are a number of drugs which are used to stimulate pancreatic function but often the most effective way to treat NIDDM is by diet and lifestyle changes: lose weight, take more exercise, do some form of relaxation such as yoga or meditation (stress is recognised to have a surprisingly dramatic effect on blood sugar levels) and improve your diet by eating lots of fresh fruits and vegetables and cutting down on processed, high fat, high sugar foods.

## Alternative approaches

Although no therapy has yet been found to reverse total pancreatic failure, a number of therapies can help to stimulate pancreatic function and promote general health.

Traditional Chinese medicine sees diabetes as a major imbalance in the body's energies and will focus on restoring harmony within the system and thus addressing the disease.

All the stress relieving, toning therapies (the many forms of yoga, meditation, massage, aromatherapy and reflexology) will be helpful in reducing stress and improving the general health of your body – and many have the advantage that you can do them at home whenever you have the time or inclination.

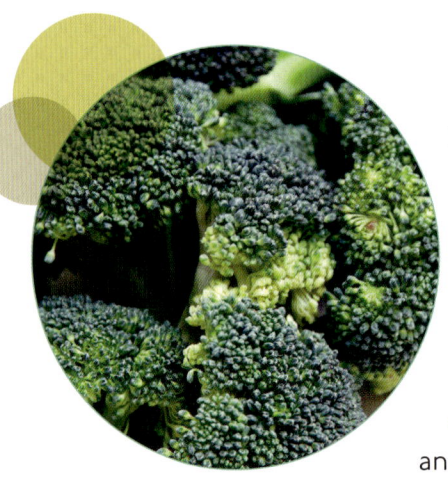

A number of foods and herbs are helpful in stimulating pancreatic function and improving blood sugar control. I have included many of the foods in the recipes that follow but here is a brief list of foods and herbs that can be beneficial to include in your daily regime:

- Whole oats, wholegrain cereals and wheat germ
- Nuts and seeds, especially walnuts, pumpkin and sunflower seeds
- All cruciferous vegetables – broccoli, cauliflower, Brussels sprouts, kale, cabbage, and bok choy
- Onions, globe artichokes and red peppers
- Lean meat and fish
- All pulses
- Sweet potatoes
- Blueberries
- Nettle and dandelion juice
- Bitter Gourd (*Momordica Charantia*)
- Cinnamon
- Garlic
- Ginseng (*Panax*)
- Hawthorn
- Pycnogenol
- Saw Palmetto
- Stevia
- Turmeric

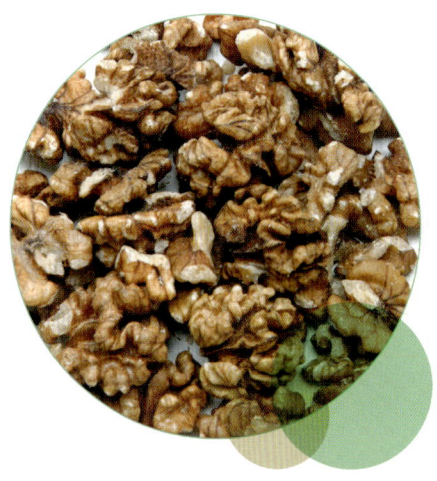

## Nutritional therapy

One of the side effects of poor blood sugar control, and the lifestyle that often leads to NIDDM, is that the person concerned has become nutrient deficient so improving one's nutritional profile can only help general health.

While a broad spectrum vitamin and mineral supplement would be good there are specific nutrients which are helpful in blood sugar control.

Chromium is an essential trace element and although we only need very little of it, it is required for the proper action of insulin. It is hard to absorb as a supplement but is available from brewer's yeast, black pepper, calves' liver, wheat germ, wholemeal bread and cheese.

Zinc, magnesium, manganese and potassium are all very important for diabetics as they are depleted through excess urination.

All the B Vitamins but especially Vitamins B6 and B12 can help blood sugar control and can be depleted by diabetic drugs. Food sources are lean meat and dairy produce.

Vitamin C strengthens fragile blood capillaries so it very helpful for diabetics as are Vitamins D3, E and K1.

Essential fatty acids, especially Omega 3 fatty acids, are important for diabetics as their absorption from normal sources may be impeded by high blood sugars.

Other useful supplements are Lipoic acid and L-Arginine.

## Blood sugar control: hyper and hypoglycaemia

The most important thing for any diabetic is to keep their blood sugar levels 'normal' thus avoiding the long term consequences of elevated blood sugar levels. However, there are also consequences to allowing your blood sugars to fall too low – and much more obvious and dramatic ones than letting them get too high.

A diabetic therefore, needs to remain continually aware of his or her blood sugars. This is **not** to say that they need to become obsessed by it, but that they need to take control of it, rather than letting it take control of them.

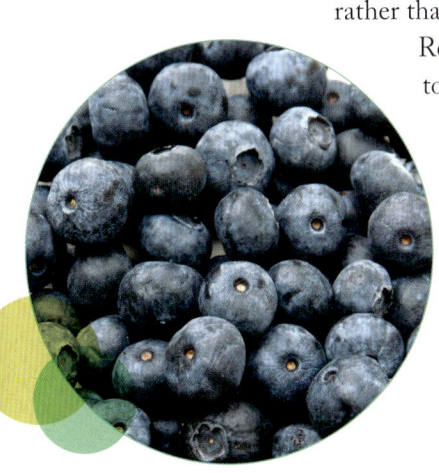

Regular testing of blood sugar levels (it takes only 30 seconds to do) will allow them to adjust their insulin levels (if they are IMMD) and their food intake/exercise to maintain relatively normal blood sugar levels and therefore be able to live a perfectly healthy and 'normal' life. The best controlled diabetics I know test four or five times a day and before every meal.

However, none of us are perfect and occasionally even the most careful diabetic will suffer from hyperglycaemia (high blood sugar) or hypoglycaemia (low blood sugar).

## Hyperglycaemia

You will probably only be aware that your blood sugars are raised when you test but remember that over eating, not taking as much exercise as usual, forgetting to take you medication, excess stress or illness may all raise your blood sugars.

## Hypoglycaemia – usually only relevant to IMMD

Hypoglycaemia occurs when the blood sugars fall too low – under 3mmol/litre. This normally happens if too much insulin has been taken in relation to the amount of food eaten or the amount of exercise taken.

Since the body is effectively being starved of energy/glucose it will, quite rapidly, cease to function properly. Symptoms vary but, since the brain is the first organ to react to a lack of fuel, they include, initially, brain fog, lack of concentration, a feeling that you must finish what you are doing before taking any medication (very dangerous if you are driving a car) and violent mood changes. This can be followed by poor coordination (so that you may stagger and look drunk) and eventually, will cause the diabetic to lose consciousness.

Although the symptoms sound (and indeed can be) dramatic, the treatment is incredibly simple – eating some sugar (glucose tablet, lumps of sugar, honey, sweets, fruit juice, sweet biscuit etc). The effect will be almost immediate – but certainly within minutes. However, the initial injection of sugar will be quickly used so needs to be followed by some more substantial food to normalise the system.

It is because of these dramatic symptoms that that it is very important that insulin dependent diabetics tell their friends that they are diabetic (and what to do if they should suffer from a hypo) and wear some sort of medical identification. If they are suffering from a severe hypo they will not be able to treat themselves and will need someone else to intervene and feed them their life-reviving glucose.

It is also very important that insulin dependent diabetics should ensure that in every trouser pocket, every jacket pocket, every handbag, in the glove pocket of their car, their golf bag, their sports bag….. they keep a few glucose tablets or sweets so that they can immediately take action if they feel a hypo coming on – and so that anyone trying to help them can find them an immediate source of sugar.

# Diet

Whatever other measures you may take to manage your diabetes, the bedrock of your treatment should be managing your diet. This does not mean, thank goodness, having to follow the horrendously complicated system of 'exchanges' that our parents and grandparents had to deal with, but it does mean being aware of what you eat, how much of it you eat and, if you are insulin dependent, when you eat it.

It will also mean, if your diet up till now has been heavily dependent on processed foods, changing the way you eat. But although this may involve some more work in cooking terms, for relatively little extra effort you will end up with a much more delicious, much healthier – and a quite possibly cheaper – diet than you had before. And just to reassure you – I am a

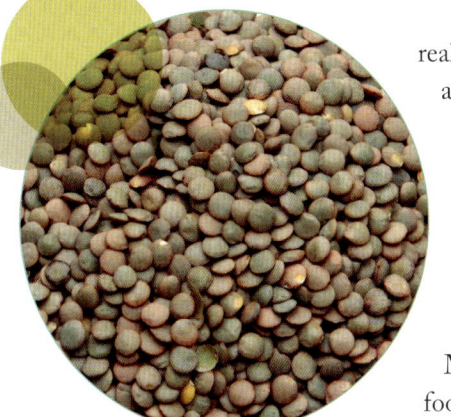

really lazy cook, so none of the recipes in this book need any more input than is absolutely necessary.

## Glycaemic Index and Glycaemic Load

In the 1990s a new way of measuring the blood-sugar-raising potential of foods was developed in the US by a NIDDM, Type 2 diabetes sufferer called David Mendosa. The Glycaemix Index ranked individual foods by how fast they broke down and turned into sugar/glucose in the body. Thus sugar has a Glycaemic Index of 100 (as it converts instantly) whereas kidney beans have an index of 40 and cherries have an index of 22, etc.

However, the GI only told you how fast a particular food turned into sugar – which made for a lot of complicated calculations if you wanted to use it as a way of assessing the suitability of a food. The system was therefore refined into what is now called the Glycaemic Load which assesses each food in the context of a serving size thus allowing you quite easily to tot up the total Glycaemic Load you would be eating in a day and thereby keep below the recommended maximum which is usually set at around 500.

In the notes to the recipes which follow I do quite often refer to the GL of the food but this is only as an indication as to whether the food is one that you can eat freely or should be restricting. It is a useful yardstick but I do not think that you should feel that you have to stick too rigidly to it. All other considerations aside, each person metabolises food at a different rate so although GL figures are a useful guide, they may not be totally accurate for you.

The Glycaemic Index of pasta made from wheat (most pasta) depends a lot upon the shape of the pasta (the thicker, the lower the GI), and the way it is cooked. When cooked as the Italians do, *al dente* – somewhat firm – it has the lowest Glycaemic Index. The longer you cook it, the softer it is, and the higher the GI. With variation depending upon these factors, most of the studies of wheat pasta show GIs in the 40s to low 60s, with a few dipping into the 30s.

Pasta has a low GI because of the physical entrapment of ungelatinised starch granules in a sponge-like network of protein (gluten) molecules in the pasta dough. Pasta is unique in this regard. As a result, pastas of any shape and size have a fairly low GI (30-60). Asian noodles such as hokkein, udon and rice vermicelli also have low to intermediate GI values.

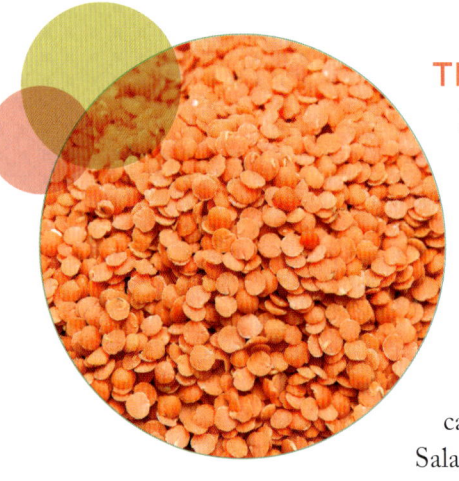

## The good, the bad and the ugly

If you would rather just work from what we know to be 'good' and 'bad' foods for diabetics, here is a short list which should give you some general guidance.

### 'Good' foods of which you can eat as much as you like

All green leafy vegetables
All cruciferous vegetables (cauliflower, broccoli, turnip, cabbage etc)
Salad vegetables
All the onion family
Green peas and beans
All mushrooms
Redcurrants, cranberries, loganberries, blueberries
Tea, coffee and water

### 'Good' carbohydrate and protein foods –
but if you are following a Glycaemic Load type diet you need to count them in as part of your daily allocation

All pulses
Brown rice and wholemeal pasta
Oats, wholemeal flours, breads and savoury crackers
All root vegetables
All other fresh fruits
Dried fruits
Unsweetened high fibre breakfast cereals
Fresh and frozen meat and fish
Cheese and yogurt
Soya products

### 'Bad-ish' foods – OK to have now and then but not to eat to excess

Refined white flour breads, pastry, rice, pasta and unsweetened biscuits
Cornflour, arrowroot
Unsweetened 'normal' breakfast cereals
Any fried or deep fried foods such as chips and crisps
Fatty and salty meat and fish products – such as sausages or salami
Fruit juices

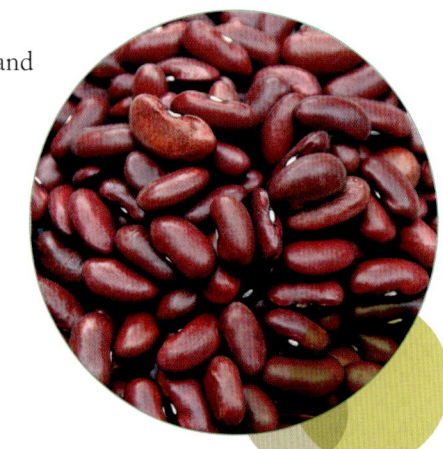

Reduced sugar jams and marmalades
Alcohol

### 'Ugly' foods – to be avoided whenever possible and only ever consumed in small quantities

All sugars, honey and golden syrup
All sweets and confectionery
Full sugar chewing gum
Full sugar jams, marmalades etc
Ice creams and ice lollies
Sweet biscuits and cakes, especially if made with refined white flours
Desserts, especially if made with refined white flours
Fruit canned in syrup, and all fruit squashes and sweetened drinks
Sweetened breakfast cereals

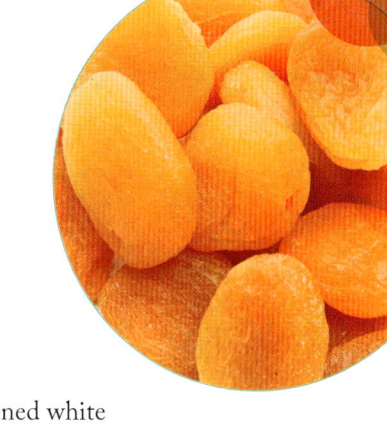

## Alcohol

Red wine, on the whole, has little effect on blood sugars (for some people it actually has a positive effect) so is probably the best drink to go for, especially as, if you are going to drink alcohol, red wine is also the best to drink if you are at risk of a heart attack or stroke.

While lager is relatively diabetic friendly, beers tend to be less so, as do spirits – and avoid liqueurs like the plague.

Also beware of low alcohol drinks as less of the sugar will have been converted into alcohol.

If you are going to use mixers, make sure they are low calorie as they will also have less sugar.

## Alternative sweeteners

I tend not to use alternative sweeteners at all in my diabetic cooking, preferring to use fresh fruits or very moderate amounts of sugar and natural sweeteners as I think they give a better flavour and, in any case, I prefer to use 'real' food. Moreover, sweeteners such as lactitol, sorbitol, maltitol can upset the digestion and cause diarrhoea.

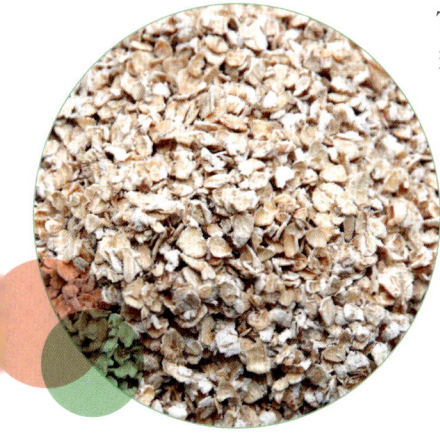

That said, Xylitol has had a very good press, is widely used in products such as toothpaste, and is very easy to use as it has roughly the same amount of sweetness as sugar.

Both the food industry and the natural health lobby have got very excited about fructose as an alternative sweetener as it is very low on the Glycaemic Index. The food industry uses it mainly as High Fructose Corn Syrup, natural foodies use it as fruit based syrups, such as agave syrup etc. But…

INTRODUCTION    15

Unlike glucose, fructose is not controlled by insulin and can only be processed by the liver.

Moreover, unlike glucose, eating fructose does not suppress the release of the stomach hormone, ghrelin. Ghrelin is the hormone that makes you feel hungry, so, if it is not suppressed when you eat, you are going to go on feeling hungry and go on eating fructose-sweetened foods whereas you might have stopped eating glucose-sweetened foods because you felt full.

And strangely, although it is a carbohydrate (therefore a sugar) fructose is processed by the liver as a fat so, rather than being stored in the liver as harmless glycogen, it gets stored as potentially harmful fat. Thus excess fructose consumption leads to excess fat being stored in the liver which can cause inflammation (with all its attendant ills) and liver disease.

So, far from fructose helping diabetics keep their weight down, it might well add to their risk of obesity, heart disease, stroke etc.

## The Recipes

The recipes which follow are designed for one or two people but can easily be scaled up if you are entertaining – but remember to 'scale up' ingredients such as cooking oil and seasoning slightly less than the main ingredients. I hope that all the dishes will be good enough for you to want to eat them again so, even if you are on your own, two helpings will be welcome as you can always freeze the remaining portion.

All are for dishes which could be eaten by anyone, diabetic or not – and many would be suitable, with a minimum of adjustment, for those with other dietary restrictions such as gluten or dairy.

All are made from 'real' food, none are either lengthy or complicated and all are designed to encourage you to cook and experiment on your own thus making cooking for a diabetic diet an exciting voyage of discovery rather than a chore. I hope you enjoy them….

# SOUPS AND STARTERS

CARROT AND RED LENTIL SOUP

CELERIAC SOUP WITH SMOKED MACKEREL

LEEK AND FENNEL SOUP

SMOKED HADDOCK CHOWDER

KIDNEY SOUP

WATERCRESS SOUP

SALAMI AND OKRA SAVOURY

AJWAR

CREAM OF MUSHROOM SOUP

# CARROT AND RED LENTIL SOUP

A North African soup with lots of flavour. The crumbled bacon adds an extra dimension – although it strays somewhat from the soup's ethnic origins! If you prefer it to be vegetarian, a squeeze of lemon juice and a few leaves of parsley will be just perfect. | Serves 2

---

1 tbsp olive oil

1 large clove garlic, peeled and sliced

1 level tsp ground cumin

¼ level tsp ground coriander

125g/5oz carrots, scrubbed and sliced

100g/4oz red lentils

450ml/15floz vegetable stock

sea salt and freshly ground black pepper

juice ½ -1 lemon

2 rashers bacon, chopped small and briskly fried till crisp (optional)

few leaves of parsley (optional)

---

Heat the oil in a medium-sized, heavy pan and add the garlic, cumin and coriander. Stir and cook for a minute or two taking great care that it does not burn.

Add the carrots and continue to cook gently for a further 5 minutes.

Add the lentils and the stock, bring to the boil, cover and simmer for 35-40 minutes or until the carrots are quite cooked.

Purée in a processor or liquidiser and adjust the seasoning to taste.

To serve, reheat, add lemon juice to taste and sprinkle with the bacon bits or chopped parsley.

*Despite the fact that both carrots and lentils feel starchy and filling, they are both low Glycaemic Load so you can enjoy this soup with a totally clear conscience.*

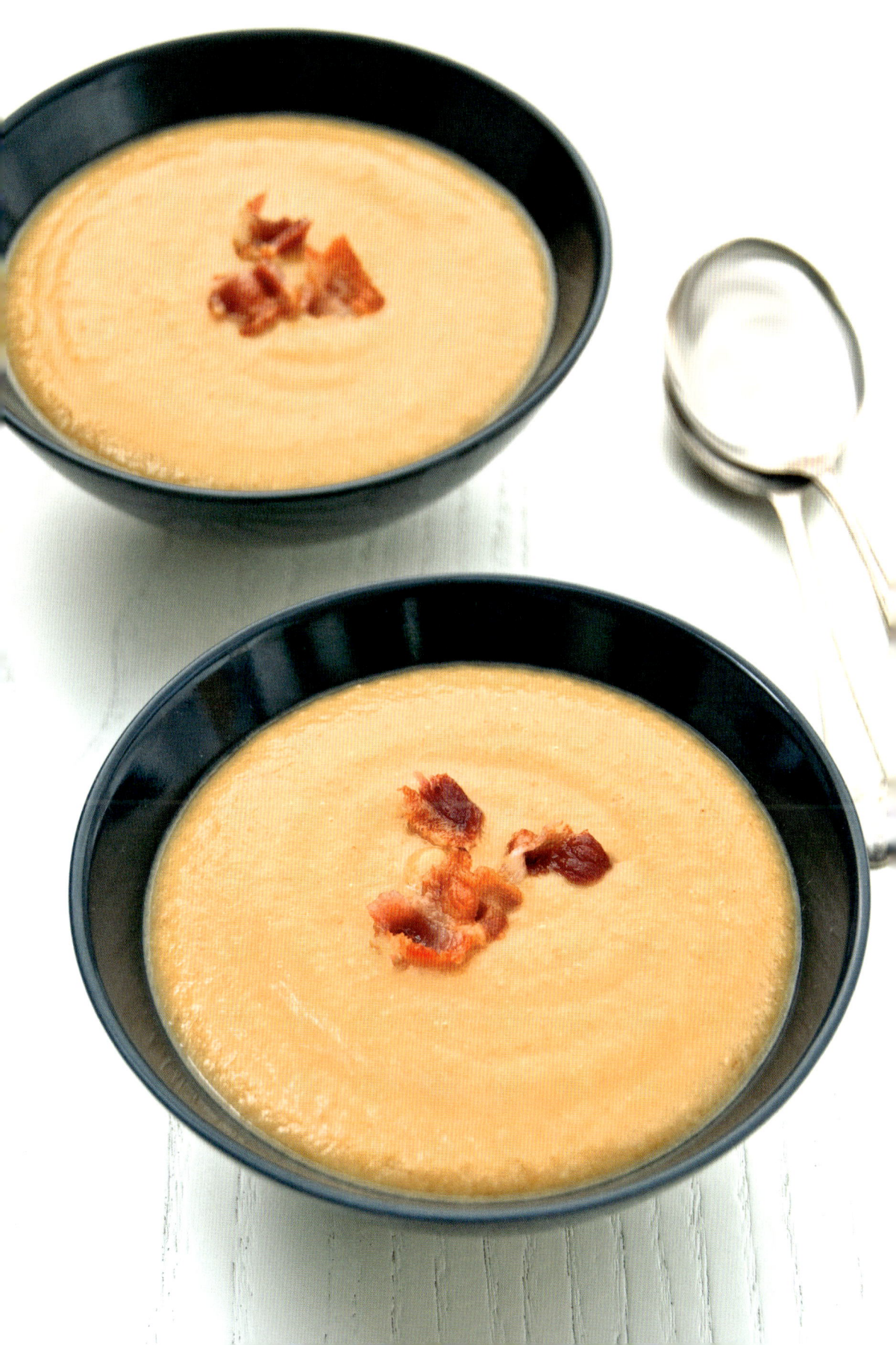

# CELERIAC SOUP WITH SMOKED MACKEREL

You can make this soup with the celeriac alone and, even though its ingredients are so simple, it is really delicious. The smoked mackerel gives it a little edge – and turns it into a full meal.
| Serves 2

---

1 medium onion
250g/9oz celeriac
400ml/14floz vegetable stock
6 tbsp milk – cow, soya or oat, as you prefer
25-50g/1-2oz smoked mackerel fillets, peppered or not,
depending on how substantial you want your soup to be
sea salt and freshly ground black pepper

---

Peel and chop the onion and put it in a pan. Scrub the celeriac and peel off any earthy or green portions; cut into large dice and add to the pan.

Add the stock, bring to the boil and simmer for 30-40 minutes or until the celeriac is quite soft.

Purée in a food processor, then add the milk and mix well. Season lightly – especially if you are using peppered mackerel.

Break the mackerel into very small pieces and add to the soup, keeping back just enough to decorate each bowl. To serve, reheat gently but do not boil. Adjust seasoning to taste and serve with a few little bits of smoked mackerel scattered over the soup.

*Smoked mackerel is so rich and flavoursome that it really can turn a bowl of soup into a full meal. It also keeps well in the fridge and is great in sandwiches or salads – and of course it boosts your intake of oily fish, which has to be good.*

# LEEK AND FENNEL SOUP

A very simple, fresh-tasting soup. If you want to make it rather more substantial you can add a handful of pearl barley or even brown rice. | Serves 2

1 generous tbsp olive oil
2 small leeks, trimmed and thinly sliced
2 small heads fennel, trimmed and very finely sliced
500ml/17floz rice or soya-based miso
25g/1oz pearl barley or brown rice (optional)
sea salt and freshly ground black pepper
2 handfuls of baby spinach leaves
a few extra slices of fennel to decorate

Heat the oil in a heavy pan and add the leeks and fennel.

Cook very gently for 10 minutes, then cover and sweat for a further 30-40 minutes.

If you are using it, add the pearl barley or rice.

Add the miso, bring to the boil, cover and reduce to a simmer for a further 30-40 minutes.

Season to taste before serving (the miso can be quite salty).

Add the spinach leaves at the same time as the seasoning and allow them to wilt in the heat of the soup.

Serve decorated with a few extra slices of fennel.

> Miso is the traditional Japanese 'stock' which is made from fermented soya beans, rice or barley mixed with salt and fungus. There are hundreds of different varieties and it is used in cooking, as a soup (a staple of Japanese daily eating), in pickles and even in some sweet dishes. Apart from being deliciously flavoursome it is also very nutritious with high levels of zinc, manganese and copper and loads of protein – 2 grams for just 25 calories. However, it is also high in salt so when using miso, do not add extra salt until you have tasted the dish.

# SMOKED HADDOCK CHOWDER

Although this chowder is a soup, it is so substantial that you can use it as a full meal. It tastes even better if you can make it a day in advance so that the flavours have time to mature.
| Serves 2

½ small leek, trimmed and sliced
2 small new potatoes, halved or sliced
50g/2oz celeriac, cut into small cubes
1 cloves of garlic, peeled and sliced
1 slice lemon
600ml/1 pint water
4 tbsp dry white wine
100g/4oz smoked haddock fillets, skinned and cut into pieces
1 fresh tomato, skinned and chopped
1 handful of dried, mixed seaweeds
sea salt and freshly ground black pepper

Put the leeks, potatoes, celeriac, garlic and lemon in a wide pan with two-thirds of the water and the wine. Bring to the boil and simmer briskly, uncovered, for 20-30 minutes or until the vegetables are cooked.

Add the smoked haddock and tomatoes and cook for a further 10 minutes. The liquid should be quite reduced.

Add the remaining water plus the sea vegetables, bring back to the boil and continue to cook for a further 15 minutes.

Season to taste if necessary (the seaweed may be enough) before serving.

Seaweeds, a staple of Japanese cooking, are very tasty, highly nutritious and have a negligible Glycaemic Load so are a great addition to any soup or salad, especially one which already contains fish. You can buy mixed packs of dried seaweeds or sea vegetables in most good delicatessens or health food stores. Try using them as an alternative to your usual seasoning.

# KIDNEY SOUP

Meat soups are rarely served these days, which is a shame as they make a wonderfully sustaining, healthy, warming – and delicious – meal. | Serves 2

---

2 tbsp olive oil
½ medium red onion, finely sliced
2 cloves garlic, finely sliced
4 chestnut mushrooms, finely sliced
2 lamb's kidneys, trimmed and diced
6 tbsp red wine
500ml/17floz water, chicken or vegetable stock or soya/rice miso
sea salt and freshly ground black pepper
½ tsp flour
4 tbsp medium sherry
small handful chopped curly parsley

---

Heat the oil in a pan and add the onions, garlic and mushrooms.

Cook gently for 5 minutes or until the onions are starting to soften.

Add the kidneys, cover and continue to sweat gently for a further 10 minutes. Add the red wine and the water or stock and a little seasoning, bring back to the boil, cover and simmer for 30 minutes.

Depending on whether you like your soup 'bitty' or smooth, remove 1 tbsp of the kidney mixture and purée the rest – or purée all the mixture. For a really smooth soup you will also need to sieve it.

Return to the pan (with the bits). In a small bowl make a purée with the flour and a little hot liquid. Add this to the soup.

Stir well, bring back to the boil and simmer for a few minutes to thicken slightly. Add the sherry, adjust the seasoning to taste and serve with lots of chopped parsley.

Offal is a sadly under-rated food – 'Oh yuck, that's gross' is all too often the reception it gets. Yet, although the texture may not appeal to all, if used in, for example, a soup, texture ceases to be an issue while the nutrition factor remains extremely high. Lamb's kidneys, for example, while having a minimal Glycaemic Load, are an excellent source of protein, thiamin, riboflavin, niacin, vitamin B12, pantothenic acid, iron, phosphorus, copper and selenium and a good source of vitamins B6 and C and zinc.

# WATERCRESS SOUP

Traditionally, watercress soup is thickened with potatoes – so, to be different I thought I would thicken mine with flageolet beans – which also just happen to be very low on the Glycaemic Index. It can be served hot or cold. | Serves 2

---

½ head fennel
2 bunches fresh watercress
500ml/17floz vegetable stock
200g tin flageolet beans
sea salt and freshly ground black pepper
1 tbsp pine nuts or sunflower seeds (optional)

---

Trim and chop the fennel and put it in a large pan.

If you are serving the soup cold, reserve a few leaves for decoration then trim the thickest stalks off the watercress and add to the fennel along with the stock.

Bring to the boil and simmer for 20 minutes, then add the beans and continue to simmer for a further 10 minutes.

Meanwhile toast the pine nuts or sunflower seeds under the grill or in a dry frying pan until lightly tanned.

Purée the soup in a food processor then return to the pan and season to taste. If you wish to serve it hot, reheat and serve sprinkled with the pine nuts or seeds.

If you wish to serve it cold, chill for a couple of hours then serve decorated with the remaining watercress leaves.

*Watercress is usually used just in salads, soup being about the only occasion on which it is cooked. However, this is a shame as it has a great flavour and nutritional profile and is an excellent addition to cooked dishes, especially egg dishes such as omelettes or frittatas.*

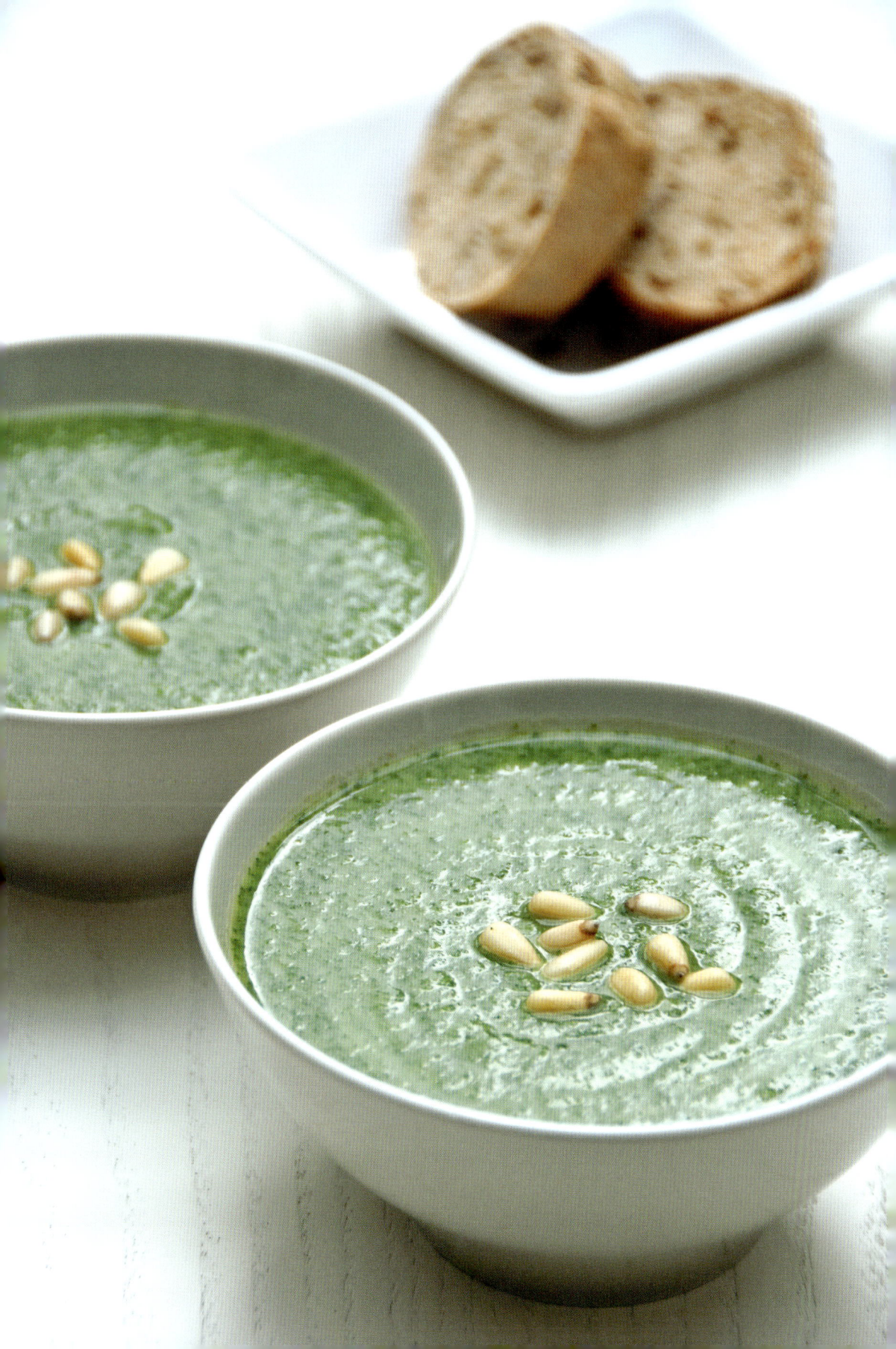

# SALAMI AND OKRA SAVOURY

This is a delicious little bonne bouche which you could have as a starter – or pile it on toast and have it for lunch. | Serves 1 (double quantities for 2)

3 slices of salami of your choice
3 pieces of okra, uncooked
1 spring onion
½ tbsp cider vinegar
1 tbsp olive oil
black pepper
4 sprigs fresh basil
4 small lettuce leaves

Cut the salami into small squares. Top the okra and slice thickly. Trim the spring onions and slice thinly horizontally.

Mix all together in a bowl and dress with the vinegar, oil and black pepper – the salami will probably be salty enough for you not to need any extra salt.

Chop two sprigs of the basil and mix it gently in.

Lay the lettuce out on your plate and pile the salami mixture in the middle. Decorate with the remaining sprigs of basil and serve.

Alternatively, lay the lettuce leaves on a slice of wholemeal toast, then pile on the salami mixture.

Okra, which is excellent for diabetics as its gooey, mucilaginous juices are very helpful for blood sugar control, is normally served cooked but, in fact is delicious raw. Nicely crisp on the outside and soft inside, it does not taste remotely gooey and makes a great contrast to the soft salami.

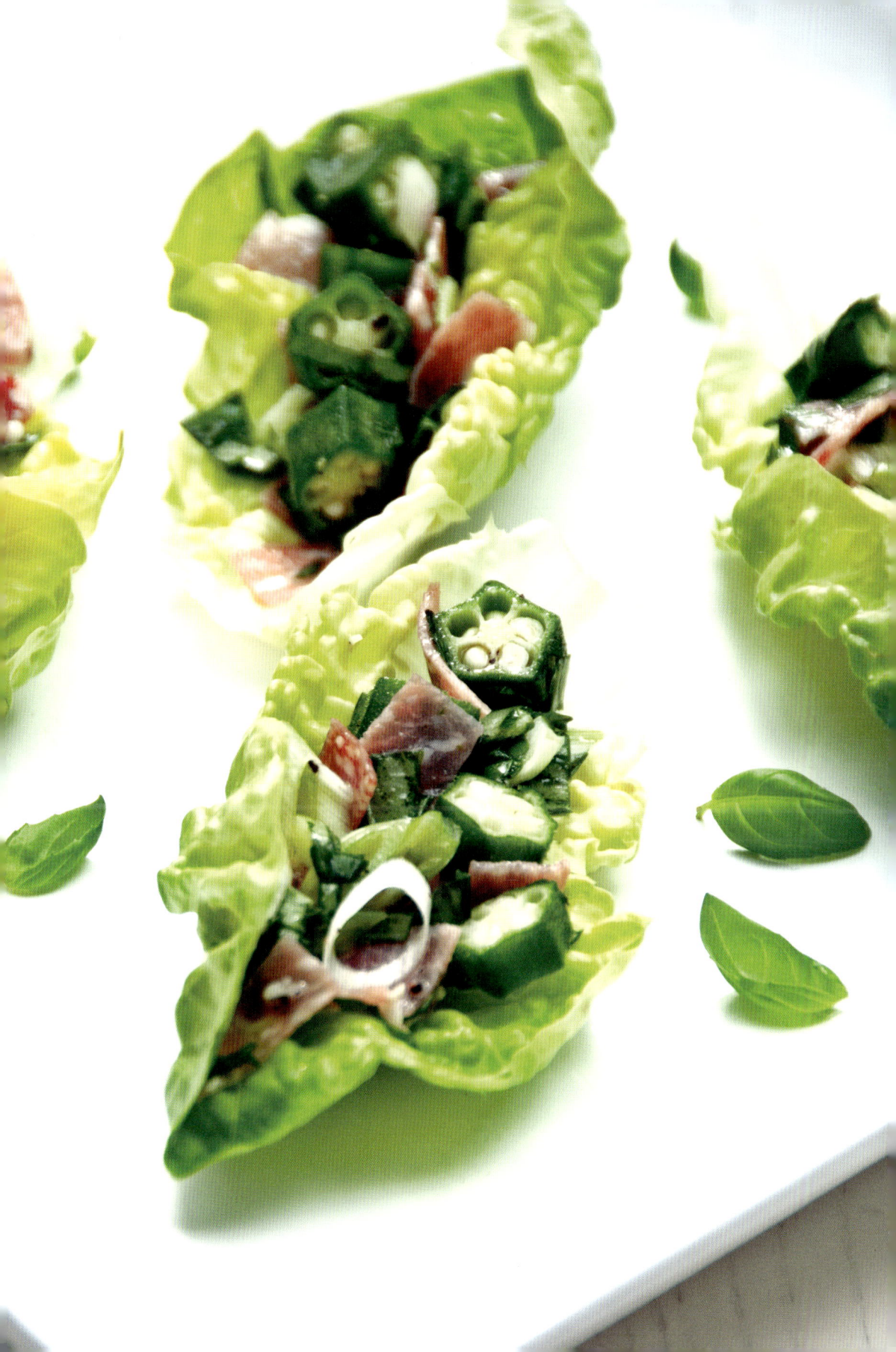

# AJWAR

Ajwar is a Yugoslavian paté made with the red peppers so beloved in south-eastern Europe. Purists will skin the peppers by submerging them in hot oil till they blister, and look askance at the addition of aubergine, let alone brown bread. However, skinning the peppers is a slow and fiddly business which I feel is scarcely justified by the marginal improvement in the flavour, and the paté is so rich in its native form that a little 'dilution' does not go amiss. It is delicious served either with fresh brown bread or toast or as a dip with crudités. It keeps well in the fridge so, even if you are on your own, it is worth making enough for 2. | Serves 2

---

2 thickish slices of aubergine

approx. 1 tbsp olive oil

1 large red pepper, deseeded and roughly chopped

1 large clove garlic

thick slice wholemeal brown bread

salt and pepper

---

Fry the aubergine slices in the oil till they are just brown on each side. Put all the ingredients – fried aubergine, peppers, garlic and bread – in a food processor and purée them.

The paté should not be totally smooth when puréed; rather it should have the texture of a country terrine.

Season lightly with salt and pepper and leave for a couple of hours for the flavours to mature then adjust the seasoning again to taste before serving with fresh brown bread, brown toast or as a dip with crudités.

> Both aubergine and peppers have negligible Glycaemic Loads so you can eat as much of this delicious paté as you want.

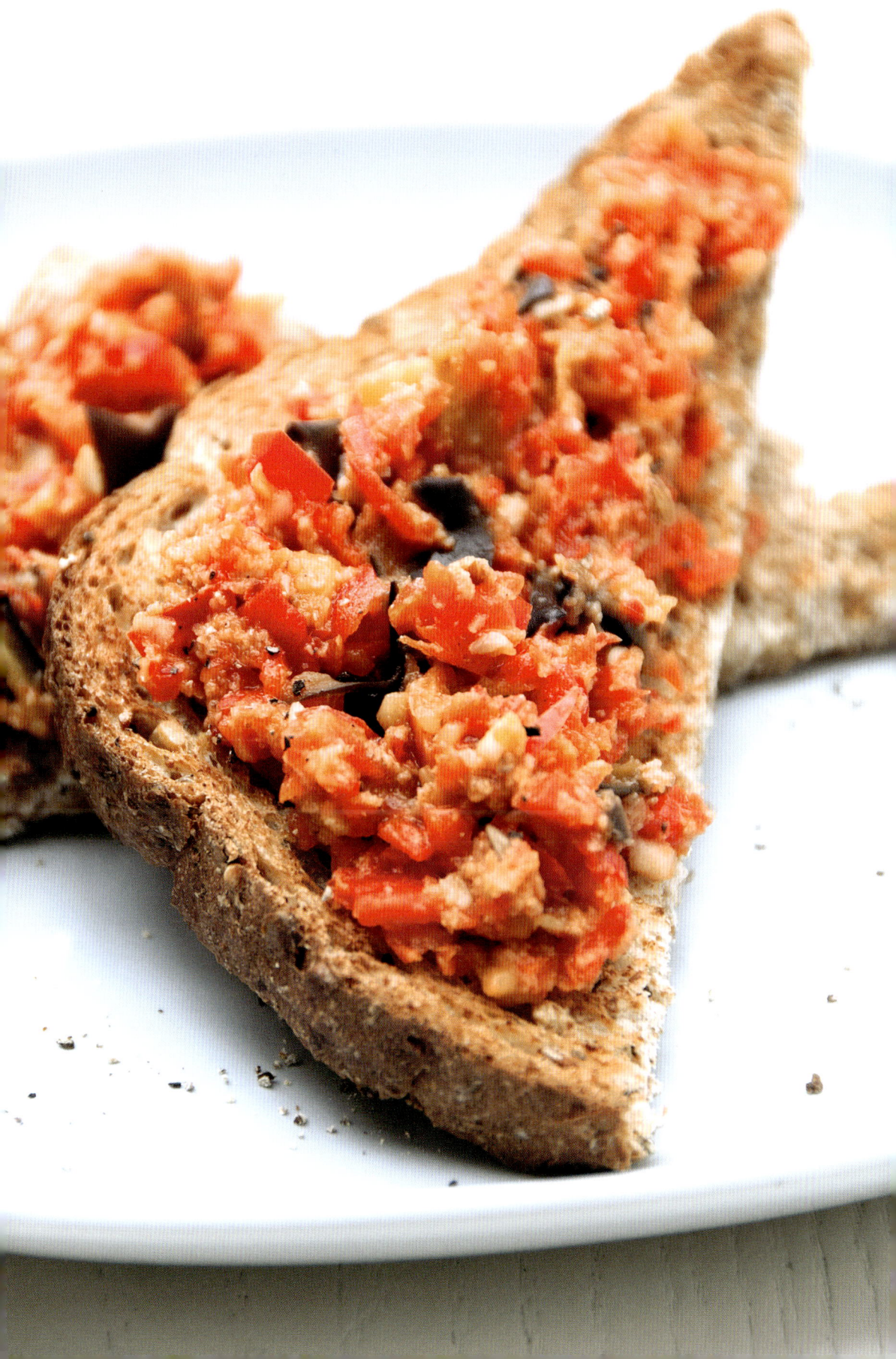

# CREAM OF MUSHROOM SOUP

A classic soup, which I always feel is improved by a hint of lemon sharpness. | Serves 2

---

1 generous tbsp olive oil
½ medium leek, sliced finely
250g/9oz chestnut mushrooms, chopped very small but not puréed
juice 1 large lemon
500ml/17floz vegetable stock
120ml/4floz cream – cow's milk, goat, oat or soya
sea salt and freshly ground black pepper
several sprigs of fresh dill weed (optional)

---

Heat the oil in a heavy pan and fry the leek gently for 4-5 minutes or until it is starting to soften. Add the mushrooms and continue to sweat gently, covered, for a further 10 minutes. Add the lemon juice and the stock, bring to the boil and simmer, covered for another 10-15 minutes.

Remove a couple of tablespoons of the mushroom bits with a slotted spoon and set aside.

Purée the rest of the soup in the food processor – how much will depend on how smooth or 'bitty' you like your soup.

Return to the pan, add the cream and season to taste, then return the extra bits of mushroom to the soup for texture.

Serve sprinkled with chopped fresh dill if you can get it.

*Mushrooms are one of those great vegetables which have, effectively, no calories, no fat, scarcely register on the Glycaemic Index yet still manage to pack a good deal of flavour and loads of nutrients including vitamin C, riboflavin, niacin, pantothenic acid, iron, phosphorus, potassium, zinc, copper, manganese and selenium.*

# EGGS

SPINACH SOUFFLÉ
LENTIL AND EGG PIE
HERB FRITTATA
EGGS AU MIROIR
HARD-BOILED EGGS WITH SPINACH

# SPINACH SOUFFLÉ

Soufflés are always regarded with great trepidation but they are really very easy to make – and the perfect meal for one or two people. As long as you remember to allow one extra egg white, you really cannot go wrong. Soufflés are very rich so just serve with a green salad. | Serves 2

---

25g/1oz butter

25g/1oz flour

1 small leek, trimmed and sliced very finely

150ml/¼ pint milk or 6 tbsp milk and 4 tbsp dry white wine

100g/4oz young spinach leaves, washed, well dried and chopped small

salt and pepper

3 eggs plus one extra egg white

25g/1oz blue cheese such Roquefort or Stilton

25g/1oz strong hard cheese such as Cheddar or Parmesan

1 tsp Dijon or wholegrain mustard (optional)

½ tsp sesame seeds (optional)

---

Heat the oven to 180C/350F/Gas mark 4.

Heat the butter in a small pan and gently cook the leeks until they are quite soft.

Add the spinach, cover and continue to cook gently until the spinach is quite wilted.

Add the flour, stir well and cook for a minute or two without burning then gradually add the milk or milk and wine, stirring continuously and continue to heat, stirring, until the sauce thickens.

Add the cheese and season to taste, adding the mustard if you want to use it.

Remove from the heat and stir in the egg yolks. Whisk the egg whites till they just hold their shape in soft peaks. Stir ⅓ of the whites into the spinach mixture and fold in the rest.

Pour into a small soufflé dish (it should come ¾ of the way up the dish) and sprinkle over the sesame seeds if you are using them.

Bake for 20-25 minutes or till it is risen and golden. Serve at once. The soufflé should be set on the outside but still soft in the middle.

*The same basic proportions can be used for any soufflé, sweet or savoury but be aware that the 'solider' and the 'wetter' your flavouring the more difficult it will be for the eggs to lift it. So chocolate or a liqueur in a sweet soufflé will give you a lighter mixture than apple.*

# LENTIL AND EGG PIE

This is quite a substantial dish – vaguely related to a moussaka but a good deal less trouble to make. It will keep for a couple of days in the fridge and reheat well in a microwave if you are on your own. | Serves 2

---

1 tbsp olive oil
1 medium onion, peeled and chopped finely
1 clove garlic, peeled and chopped finely
2 rashers of back bacon or 3 anchovies, chopped finely
100g/4oz field mushrooms, chopped roughly
100g/4oz Puy or black lentils
240ml/8floz vegetable stock or miso
5 tbsp red wine
sea salt and freshly ground black pepper
2 small eggs
120ml/4floz milk – cow's milk, soya or oat milk
1 handful of fresh parsley, flat or curly

---

Heat the oil in a medium-size pan and add the onions, garlic and bacon rashers or anchovies. Fry all together briskly but without burning for 8-10 minutes or until the onions are softening and colouring lightly. Add the mushrooms and continue to cook for another 3-4 minutes or until the mushrooms are quite soft.

Add the lentils, stir around for a minute or two, then add the stock and the wine and season lightly. Bring to the boil and then simmer gently for 20-30 minutes or until the lentils are quite cooked. Adjust seasoning to taste.

Meanwhile, heat the oven to 180C/350F/Gas mark 4.

Beat the eggs in a bowl with the milk and season lightly. Chop the parsley fairly finely and add to the egg mixture.

Spoon the lentils into an oven-proof casserole then pour the egg mixture over the top. Bake in the preheated oven for 25 minutes or until the egg topping is set and slightly risen and browned.

Serve at once with a green vegetable or salad.

*Lentils are low on the Glycaemic Index and have a low Glycaemic Load so are an excellent filling – and tasty – food for any diabetic.*

# HERB FRITTATA

This omelette is perfect for the summer when the herbs are all fresh. It can be eaten warm or left to cool and eaten in wedges with a salad or for a picnic. I am therefore giving quantities for two – so that even if you are only catering for one there will be plenty left for the next days' lunch. | Serves 2

---

2 tbsp olive oil

1 small leek, sliced very finely

1 clove garlic, peeled and sliced

25g/1oz fresh broad beans or fresh or frozen petits pois

1 small handful fresh spinach

1 small handful fresh watercress

2 sprigs fresh mint

2 sprigs fresh parsley

1 small handful fresh coriander (optional)

4 medium eggs

2 tbsp water

1 tbsp pine nuts

sea salt and freshly ground black pepper

25g/1oz grated Parmesan

---

Heat 1 tablespoon oil in a small frying pan and very gently cook the leeks and garlic till they are quite soft. Meanwhile steam the broad beans, if you are using them, till they are just cooked and then skin them; if you are using the petits pois, steam till just cooked but still slightly crunchy.

Chop all the herbs roughly. Beat the eggs with the water in a large bowl. Add the leeks and garlic, the beans, chopped herbs and pine nuts and season generously.

Heat your grill.

Heat a further tablespoon of oil in your frying or omelette pan till almost smoking. Pour in the egg mixture and cook briskly for a couple of minutes till the base of the omelette is firm.

Sprinkle the Parmesan over the top of the omelette and place under the hot grill to cook and brown the top of the omelette, but take care that it does not burn.

Eat at once with crusty bread.

*Fresh broad beans are a real treat if you can make the effort to skin them. This is a bit of a fiddle, but worth it. Steam them until just cooked then break the skin with a sharp knife or your finger nail and just pop the bean out. The skinless beans are a beautiful fresh green and taste delicious.*

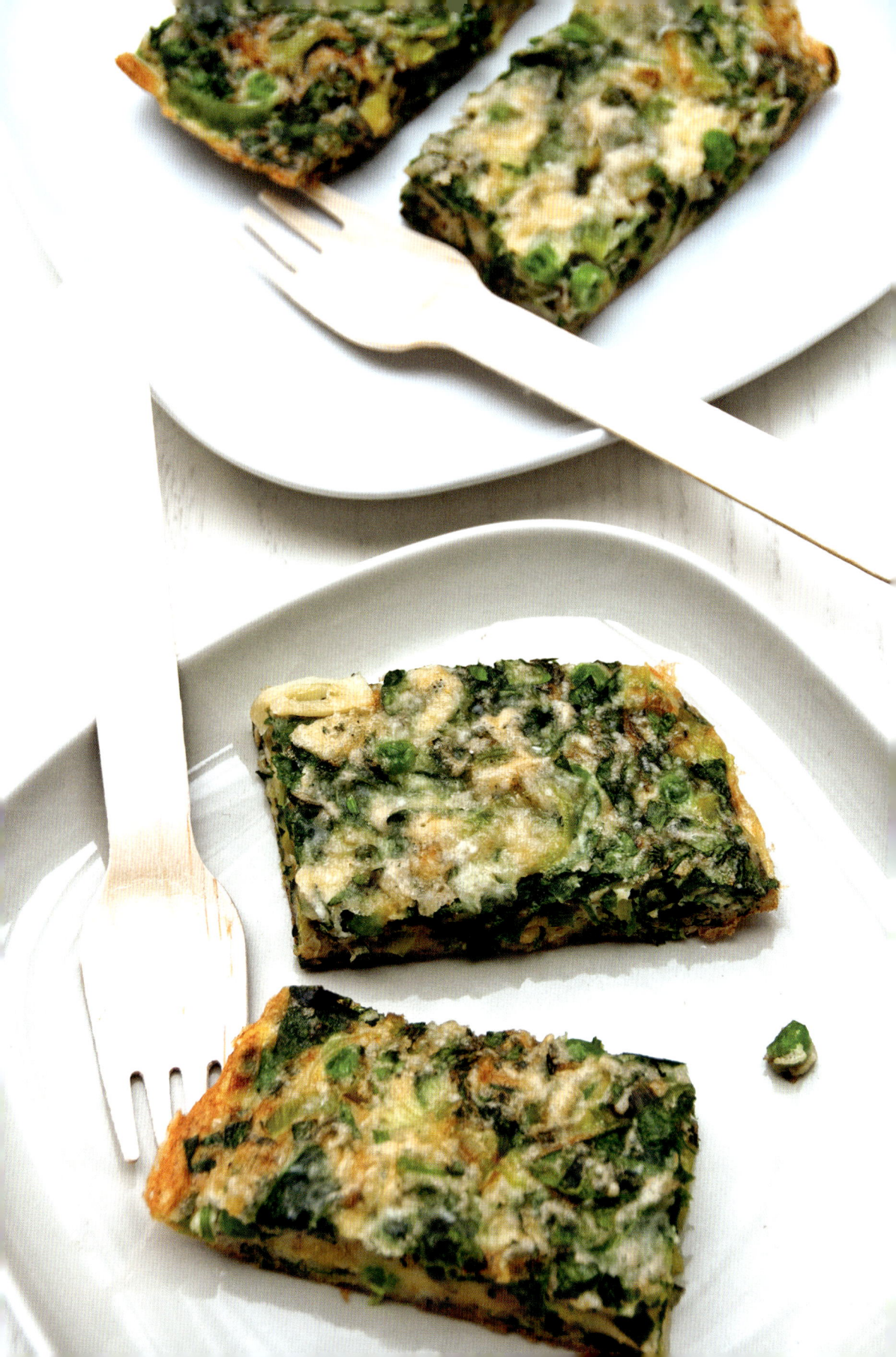

# EGGS AU MIROIR

This is a really unusual combination of flavours based on an 18th century recipe. You can use it as a starter or as a light meal. | Serves 1 (double quantities for 2)

10g/¼ oz butter
2 spring onions, finely chopped
1 tbsp finely chopped parsley
2 medium eggs
4 tbsp cream (or soya or oat cream if you wish to keep the fat levels down)
juice of ½ a small orange and ½ a small lemon
salt and white pepper

Heat the oven to 160C/325F/Gas mark 3.

Rub the bottom of a cocotte dish large enough to hold the eggs with the butter and spread the onions and parsley over it.

Carefully break the eggs into the dish. Mix the cream with the juices, season them fairly generously and pour them over the eggs. Bake for 15-20 minutes or till the whites of the eggs are just set.

Serve the eggs with brown toast or fresh brown bread, and a green salad if you are having it as a main meal.

*Eighteenth century cooks often combined orange and lemon juice with cream to achieve a rich dish which was not cloying – a very successful tactic!*

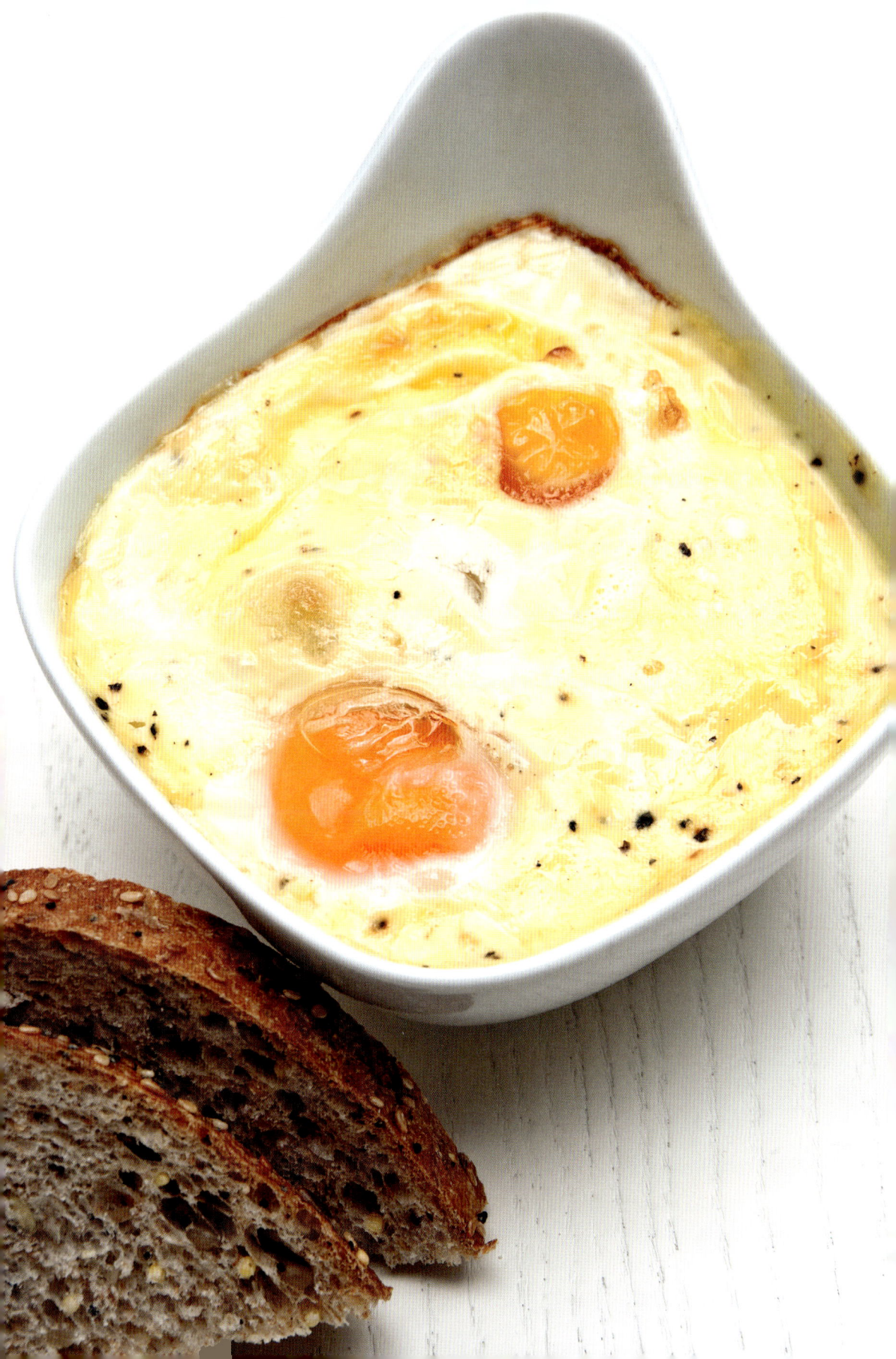

# HARD-BOILED EGGS WITH SPINACH

A very traditional combination, given a little spice by the slightly bitter chicory. | Serves 1 (double quantities for 2)

---

175g/6oz fresh spinach

1 tbsp good olive oil

sea salt, freshly ground black pepper and ground nutmeg

2 small eggs

1 tbsp goats', sheep or soya yogurt

juice 1/4 lemon

1/2 head chicory, finely chopped

small bunch of fresh chives (or spring onion tops), chopped small

---

Hard boil the eggs. When cooked, shell and slice.

Meanwhile, cook the spinach in 2cm/½ inch of water then drain thoroughly.

Stir in the olive oil and season with salt, pepper and nutmeg.

In a bowl mix the yogurt with the lemon juice and season to taste.

Mix in the chicory and chives.

Arrange the spinach on a plate with the sliced eggs in the middle. Spoon over the dressing and serve at once.

There are so few carbohydrates in spinach that they have no effect whatsoever on blood sugar – so you can eat as much of it as you like! Since it is also fat and cholesterol free but a good source of niacin, zinc, fibre, protein, vitamins A, B6, C, E, K, thiamin, riboflavin, folate, calcium, iron, magnesium, phosphorus, potassium, copper and manganese – you should eat lots of it.

# PASTA

Fusilli with capers and anchovies
Fettucine with smoked salmon and cream sauce
Warm pasta and curly kale salad with pumpkin seeds
Pasta and broccoli or cauliflower au gratin
Classic spaghetti carbonara

# FUSILLI WITH CAPERS AND ANCHOVIES

The capers and anchovies give this recipe a very hearty, Italian country cooking flavour. To complete the picture you could also add a few olives although I think that is slight overkill. The sauce works better if you cook slightly more of it so I have given the recipe for two. However, any excess will keep for several days in the fridge – and would also be excellent on toast. | Serves 2

---

1 tbsp olive oil

2/3 x 50g/2oz tin anchovies

2 shallots, peeled and chopped

2 cloves garlic, peeled and sliced

5 field mushrooms, chopped fairly roughly

150g/5oz dried fusilli

1 heaped tsp capers, roughly chopped

4 tbsp dry white wine

2 sprigs fresh parsley, chopped

sea salt and freshly ground black pepper

---

Heat the olive oil plus most of the oil from the anchovies in a small pan and add the shallots and garlic and the anchovies, finely chopped. Fry fairly gently for 4-5 minutes, then add the mushrooms. Continue to cook briskly.

Meanwhile, cook the fusilli in plenty of boiling water according to the instructions on the pack.

Add the capers and the wine to the sauce and continue to cook for a couple of minutes.

Drain the fusilli, reserving a little of the cooking water to add to the sauce.

Add the parsley and enough cooking water to make the sauce the consistency of single cream, then season to taste.

Mix gently into the fusilli and serve at once with a green salad.

> Remember that the Glycaemic Load of pasta is lower if you cook it, as the Italians do, so that it is slightly al dente, with just a tiny bit of chewiness. I have used a dried fusilli for this dish as being more suited to its robust flavours.

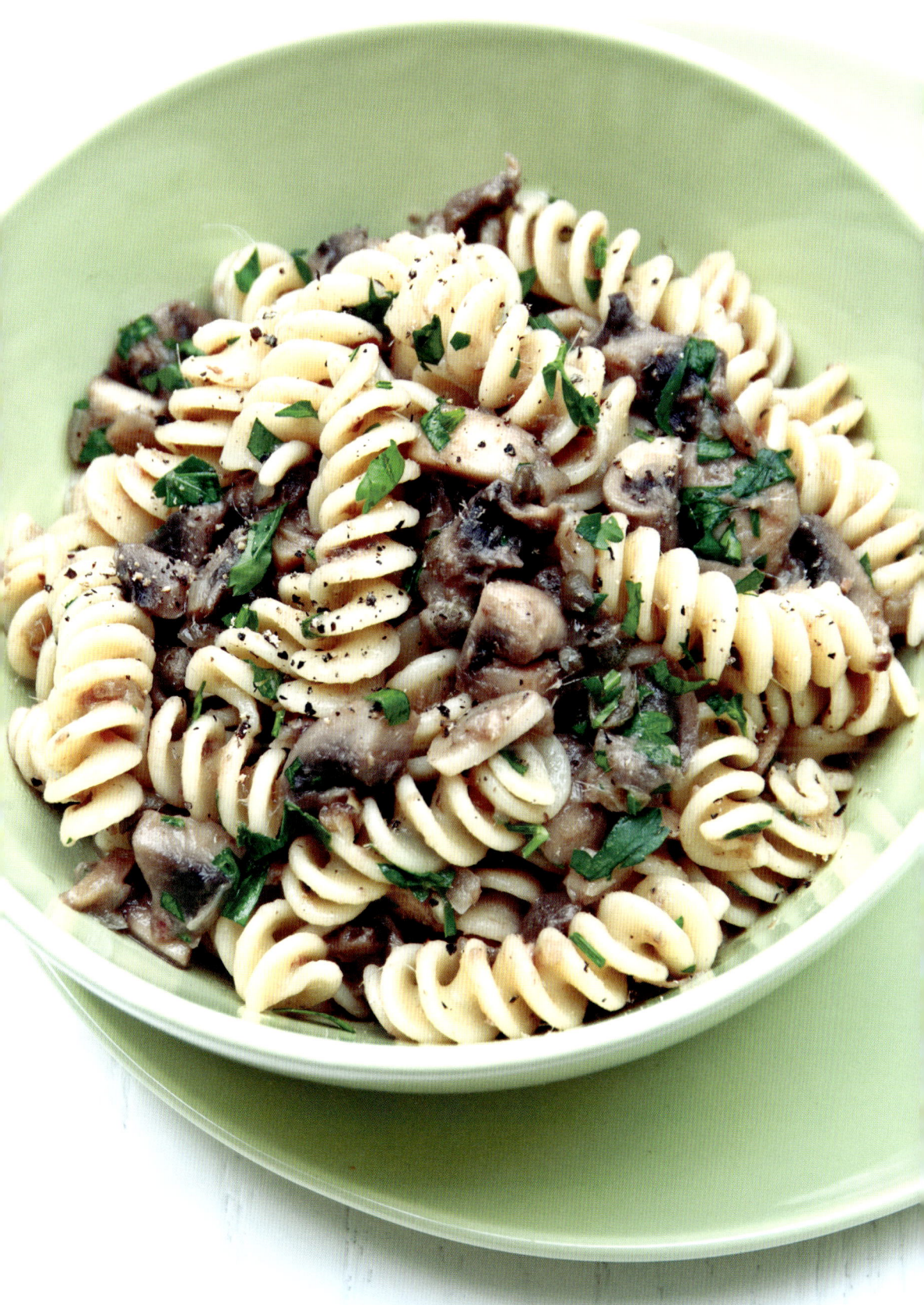

# FETTUCINE WITH SMOKED SALMON AND CREAM SAUCE

Although this looks an expensive dish, if you use the smoked salmon off-cuts to be found in most supermarkets it can actually be quite cost effective – and delicious. It is also very easy to make in single portions. Because it is relatively delicate, a fresh pasta will be better. | Serves 1 (double quantities for 2)

---

1 scant tbsp olive oil

25g/1oz button mushrooms, finely sliced

4 tbsp dry white wine

$1/2$ tsp fresh dill, chopped or scant $1/2$ tsp level tsp dried

4 tbsp single cow's milk cream or soya or oat cream

75g/3 oz smoked salmon (or salmon off-cuts) cut in matchsticks

juice $1/2$ lemon

sea salt and freshly ground black pepper

75g/3oz fresh fettucine or other ribbon pasta

---

Heat the oil in a small pan and gently fry the mushrooms for 2-3 minutes; do not let them colour. If you are using dried dill add it along with the wine, increase the heat and cook fast for a further 2 minutes to reduce the wine. Remove from the heat and add the cream and the salmon and season to taste with salt, pepper and lemon juice. Cover, set aside and keep just warm.

Cook the pasta according to the instructions on the pack till it is just *al dente*. Gently mix in the salmon sauce and, if you are using fresh dill, sprinkle it over the dish to serve.

*Soya or oat cream, both of which are low in saturated fat and cholesterol free, will taste just as good in this dish as 'normal' cream.*

# WARM PASTA AND CURLY KALE SALAD WITH PUMPKIN SEEDS

I think that pasta is often best served warm, rather than hot – which also puts less pressure on the cook. This is quite a 'hearty' dish but tasty.

You could make this with whole wheat pasta as the stronger flavour is a good match for the curly kale. | Serves 1 (double quantities for 2)

---

2 tbsp olive oil

1 small onion, peeled and sliced

4 or 5 small button mushrooms, halved or sliced

75g/3oz dried penne, whole wheat if possible

50g/2oz curly kale, trimmed of its stalks and chopped

25g/1oz pumpkin or mixed seeds, lightly toasted – you can use one of the many delicious proprietary mixes now available if you prefer

sea salt and freshly ground black pepper

juice 1/4 lemon

---

Heat 1 tablespoon of the oil in a small pan and add the onions. Cook them gently for 5-8 minutes or until they are quite soft; add the mushrooms and turn up the heat to cook more briskly for another couple of minutes or until they start to give their juice.

Meanwhile, cook the pasta in plenty of lightly salted boiling water according to the instructions on the pack. Drain and set aside.

Steam the kale for a couple of minutes only. It needs to be lightly cooked but still retain a little crunch and its greenness.

If you are using fresh seeds, toast them lightly under a grill or in a dry pan but take care not to burn them.

In a large serving dish, amalgamate the onions or mushrooms with the pasta, then add the kale and seeds.

Add the rest of the oil and season to taste with sea salt, freshly ground black pepper and the lemon juice.

Serve warm or at room temperature.

> All kinds of seeds – pumpkin, sunflower, sesame – are not only delicious but highly nutritious. However, like nuts, their flavour is really released by roasting or toasting. It only takes a minute and is well worth the effort. If you use any of the proprietary mixes (many of which are excellent) be careful when you season as a lot of them can be quite salty.

# PASTA AND BROCCOLI OR CAULIFLOWER AU GRATIN

A classic – with a twist. If I am cooking this for several people I often use both cauliflower and broccoli but if you are only cooking for one or two it might be more practical just to use one or the other – unless, of course, you happened to have some left overs in the fridge in which case it would be a great way to use them up… | Serves 1 (double quantities for 2)

---

50g/2oz dried penne or fusilli

75g/3 oz broccoli or cauliflower florets or a mixture of the two

½ small onion, chopped very roughly

15g/½oz butter

15g/½oz flour

6 tbsp milk (cow's milk, soya milk or oat milk)

2 tbsp dry white wine

50g/2oz cheese, grated – you could use a good cheddar, a strong Italian cheese such a Parmesan or a blue cheese – or a combination

1 tsp whole grain or Dijon mustard

sea salt and freshly ground black pepper

---

Cook the pasta according to the instructions on the packet, drain and keep warm reserving a little of the water to thin the sauce if needed.

Meanwhile, steam the broccoli and/or cauliflower and onions until they are just cooked but still slightly al dente.

While the pasta and vegetables are cooking, heat the butter in a pan and add the flour. Cook gently for a minute then slowly add the milk and wine and continue to heat, stirring continuously, until the sauce thickens. Add ¾ of the cheese, then season to taste. If the sauce is too thick, thin it with a little of the pasta water.

Gently mix the pasta with the vegetables, then spoon both into a warmed casserole or pie dish. Sprinkle the remaining cheese over the top and brown under a grill. Serve at once.

> Blue cheeses are very good for cooking as the heat really brings out the flavour so you need relatively less of them to achieve the same results.

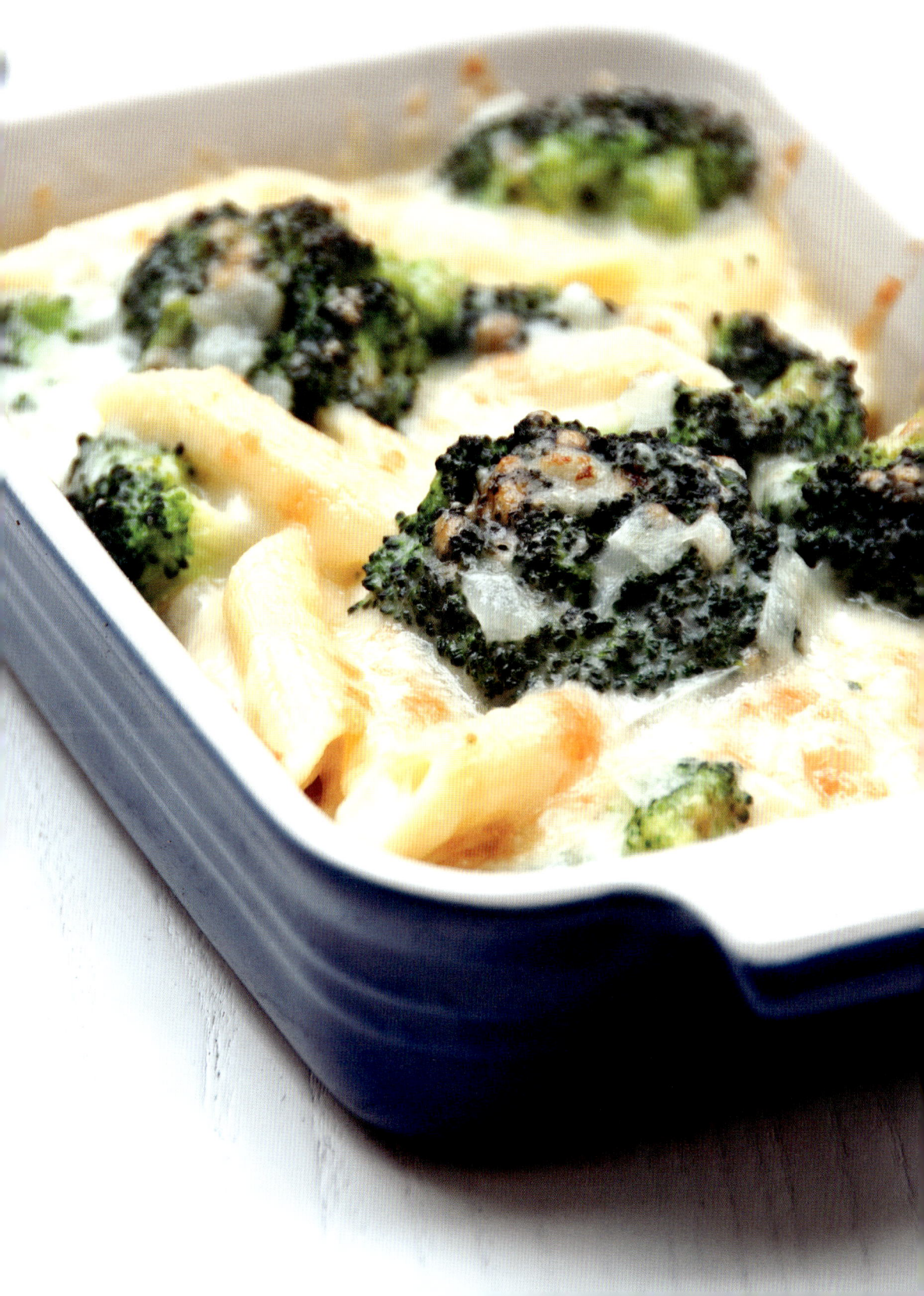

# CLASSIC SPAGHETTI CARBONARA

This is a classic but it is so easy, so quick, so tasty and so nourishing that I thought it was worth including. | Serves 1 (double quantity for 2)

---

1 tbsp olive oil
1 small onion, peeled and finely chopped
1 clove garlic, peeled and sliced
pinch salt
2-3 rashers of fatty back bacon, cut up small
100g/4oz fresh or dried spaghetti
1 medium egg
freshly ground black pepper
freshly grated Parmesan (optional)

---

Heat the oil in a small pan and add the chopped onion and garlic and a pinch of salt to draw out the liquid and stop them burning. Fry gently for 5-6 minutes or until they are soft. Remove them with a slotted spoon and set aside. Add the bacon and fry briskly in the residual oil until it is crisp.

Meanwhile, cook the spaghetti in lots of fast boiling water with a dash of oil according to the instructions on the pack.

Break the egg into a bowl and beat.

When the spaghetti is cooked, drain and return to the pan. Mix in the onion and bacon thoroughly then pour in the egg and mix well in so that it coats the pasta.

Serve at once with grated Parmesan, if you can eat it.

> Warning... You are using a raw egg in this dish although, provided the pasta is hot, it will be almost entirely cooked by the heat of the dish. However, if you are concerned you can return the pan to the heat and cook for a couple of minutes extra until the egg is cooked through – although this will change the texture of the dish as the pasta will no longer be coated in the raw egg as originally intended. But it will still be very tasty.

# SEAFOOD AND FISH

STIR FRIED PRAWNS WITH GINGER
FRESH SEAFOOD SALAD
BEETROOT AND RED CABBAGE WITH ROLLMOPS
MOULES MARINIÈRES
SALMON STEAMED WITH FENNEL AND TOMATOES
SMOKED MACKEREL WITH CURLY KALE
MACKEREL BAKED WITH APPLE
STIR FRIED TUNA WITH MANGETOUT
SMOKED HADDOCK PIE
POACHED TROUT WITH RHUBARB SAUCE
FILLETS OF COD WITH CHILLI
PEPPER, PEAR AND ANCHOVY SALAD

# STIR FRIED PRAWNS WITH GINGER

A very quick and easy, but delicious way to cook prawns – and a recipe which works well for just one person. If you want to splash out, treat yourself to fresh king or jumbo prawns – but the recipe will still be tasty if you use a few frozen prawns from the freezer. | Serves 1 (double quantities for 2)

---

1 tbsp wok or stir-fry oil

15g/½ oz piece fresh ginger, peeled and sliced into thin matchsticks

50g/2oz button mushrooms, sliced

3 spring onions

125g/5oz large, raw prawns or 100g/4oz frozen prawns, defrosted in their juice and then patted dry with kitchen paper

juice 1 lime

sea salt and freshly ground black pepper

selection of green leaves

fresh crusty brown bread

---

In a wok heat the oil and add the ginger. Cook briskly, without burning for a couple of minutes, then add the mushrooms and continue to cook for another minute.

Cut the green from the spring onions and slice it lengthways into very thin matchsticks. Slice the white into separate thin matchsticks.

Add the prawns and the white part of the spring onions and continue to cook, stirring frequently until the prawns are cooked. This will take 2-3 minutes if you are using fresh prawns, slightly less if you are using frozen as they only need to be warmed through.

Add the spring onion greens, the lime juice and season to taste. Serve immediately on a bed of leaves with some crusty bread.

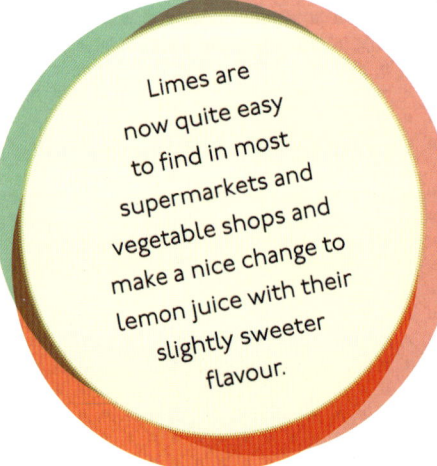

Limes are now quite easy to find in most supermarkets and vegetable shops and make a nice change to lemon juice with their slightly sweeter flavour.

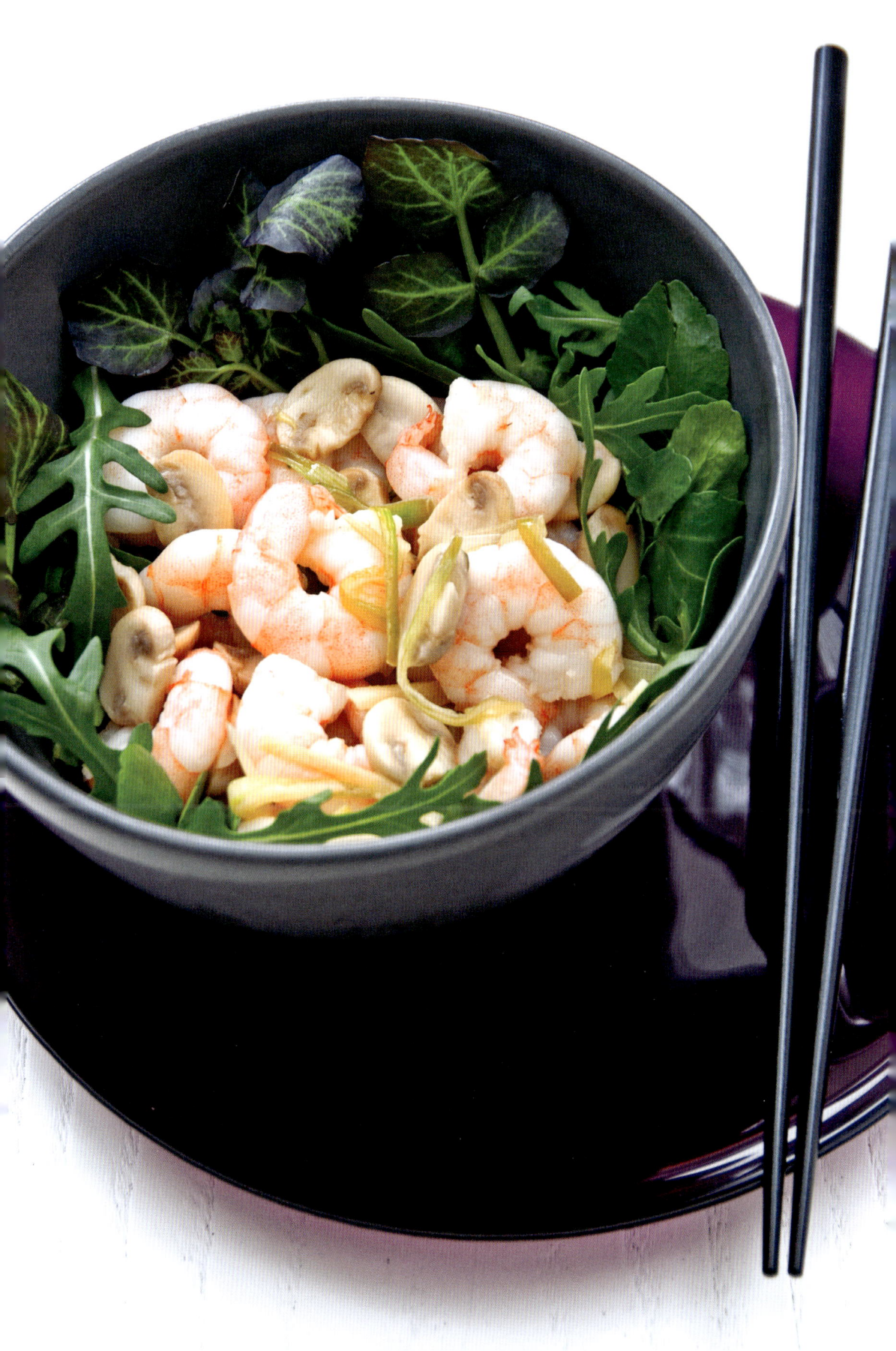

# FRESH SEAFOOD SALAD

Many supermarkets sell ready cooked mixtures of prawns, mussels, squid etc which makes this a very quick and easy dish to prepare for either one or two. Alternatively, buy 100g/4oz per person of any combination of seafood that you choose and simmer them gently in a little seasoned water mixed with a little white wine or in fish stock. | Serves 1 (double quantities for 2)

---

100g/4oz of mixed cooked seafood
1 small bulb fennel, trimmed and very finely sliced
juice of 1 lemon
2 medium tomatoes
4 young spring onions, trimmed and chopped small
¼ small mild red chilli or a generous pinch of cayenne pepper
sea salt and freshly ground black pepper
1 tbsp olive oil

---

Mix the seafood with the fennel and add the lemon juice.

Soak the tomatoes in boiling water for 1 minute then plunge them in cold water. Skin and deseed the tomatoes then cut the flesh into medium-size square and add them to the fish mixture with the spring onions.

If you are using it de-seed the chilli, slice it very thinly and then chop into tiny squares and mix gently into the fish. If using cayenne, sprinkle it over the fish then add the oil and season to taste with sea salt and black pepper.

Chill and allow to marinate for up to an hour before serving with a new potato salad and a green leaf salad.

> Chillies are another great vegetable for diabetics as it is generally accepted that they can have a significantly beneficial effect on blood sugar control – quite apart from being helpful in pain control, clearing the nose and lungs of congestion and containing significant levels of vitamins A and C, calcium, iron and potassium.

# BEETROOT AND RED CABBAGE WITH ROLLMOPS

This is what could be called a vigorous dish, with strong flavours and colours. Ideal to set you up for a long winter walk! The contrast of the warm vegetables and the cold rollmops also works well. | Serves 2

---

100g/4oz fresh beetroot, scrubbed and quartered
100g/4oz floury potatoes, scrubbed, halved and quartered
salt and freshly ground black pepper to taste
100g/4oz red cabbage, sliced thinly
½ small Bramley or other sharp cooking apple, peeled, cored and diced small
½ tsp coriander seeds, lightly crushed
4 tbsp vegetable stock or water
150ml/¼ pint plain, low fat yoghurt, cow, goat, sheep or soya
2 rollmop herrings

---

Steam the beetroot and potato for 10-15 minutes or until they are cooked, then mash and season them. Spread them in a layer in the bottom of a pie dish and keep warm.

Meanwhile put the cabbage, apple and coriander seeds in a small pan with the stock or water. Mix them well together, cover and cook gently for 5-8 minutes or until the apple is cooked through and the cabbage is cooked but still slightly crunchy. Remove from the heat and stir in ⅔ of the yogurt; spread this mixture over the mashed root vegetables.

Arrange the rollmops on top and drizzle over the rest of the yogurt. Grind over some black pepper and serve at once with crusty brown bread.

> Because of their relatively high sugar content diabetics tend to veer away from beetroot but provided they eat the whole root (and not just the juice) and combine it with other low GI foods (as in this dish), beetroots' benefits far outweigh their sugar content in nutritional terms. They are very high in vitamins A, B1, B2, B6 and C, choline, folic acid, iodine, manganese, potassium and fibre and are well known as excellent cleansers of the blood. And they taste great!

# MOULES MARINIÈRES

People tend to assume that you can only cook dishes like moules for lots of people but this is entirely wrong. It is as easy to treat yourself to a dish of moules as to treat a group – and if you are worried about that high fat, creamy sauce, you do not have to use cream. However, you do have to use fresh mussels so this is a dish for the autumn or winter when there is that 'r' in the month.

Serve with crusty brown bread to mop up the juices and a green salad to follow. | Serves 1 (double quantities for 2)

---

350g/12oz fresh mussels in their shells

15g/½oz butter

½ small onion, finely chopped

½ clove garlic, crushed

120ml/4floz dry white wine

salt and freshly ground black pepper

1 level tsp chopped parsley

---

Clean the mussels thoroughly, scraping off as many of the barnacles as possible and removing the beard (or byssus) from the pointed end. They should all close firmly when tapped, if not, throw them out; it means they are dead and must not be eaten as they will make you ill.

Heat a lidded pan large enough to hold the mussels and add the butter, onions, crushed garlic, wine and several grinds of black pepper. Bring to the simmer then add the mussels. Cover the pan, give it a good shake and simmer, with the lid on, for 5 minutes.

Warm a large bowl.

Take the mussels off the heat and, with a ladle, spoon the mussels and cooking juices into your bowl. If you pour the juices the sand which inevitably remains in the mussels goes in too.

Sprinkle over the chopped parsley and serve at once with crusty brown bread.

> Remember to wash the mussels very thoroughly and to discard any that do not close when you wash them and do not open when you cook them as that will mean that they are dead and will undoubtedly make you ill.

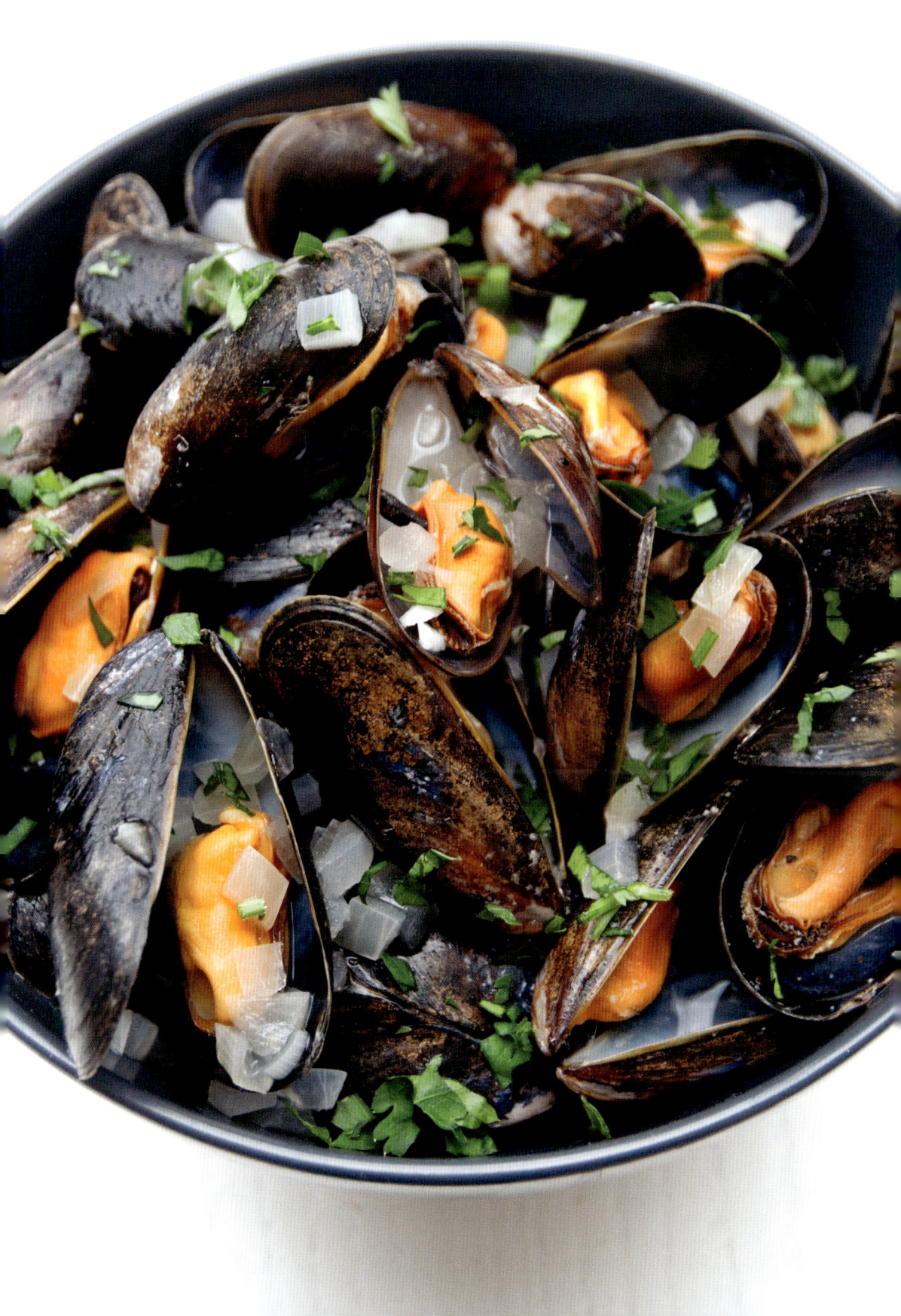

# SALMON STEAMED WITH FENNEL AND TOMATOES

If you have an electric steamer, this is the perfect dish for which to use it. If not, you can use a normal steamer or even a colander over a pan. If you can use fish stock or wine that will add flavour, but even just cooking the dish over a pan of water will be fine.

It is an 'all-in-one' dish so you should not need any extra vegetables. | Serves 1 (double quantities for 2)

---

200ml/6fl oz dry white wine, fish stock or water
75g/3oz new potatoes, scrubbed and sliced thinly
sea salt or seaweed condiment and freshly ground black pepper
1 medium tomato
½ head of fennel, sliced finely
handful of spinach leaves
1 salmon steak or cutlet
2 slices of lemon

---

Put the liquid into the lower section of your steamer.

Lay out the thinly sliced potato in the bottom of the steamer basket, overlapping the slices so that the juices from the other ingredients will not seep through. Season with sea salt or seaweed condiment and some black pepper, cover the pan and steam for 5-8 minutes or until the potatoes are starting to soften. Meanwhile, drop the tomato into a cup of boiling water for a minute, then run it under the cold tap and skin it. Slice it thinly.

Lay the fennel sliced over the potato and cover them with the sliced tomato. Season again lightly, then cover the tomato with the spinach leaves.

Lay the salmon steak or cutlet on top of the spinach and the lemon on top of the salmon.

Cover the pan and continue to steam for a further 8-9 minutes or until the salmon is cooked.

Warm a plate and carefully lift the salmon, with its bed of vegetables, out onto the plate. Grate over a little more black pepper and serve at once.

> In many ways, steaming is the ideal cooking method for a diabetic as it retains all the nutrients of the food and keeps it deliciously moist without having to use any fat at all. It is also very difficult to overcook food in a steamer – so soggy Brussels sprouts really do become a thing of the past! Electric steamers which give you two baskets so that you can steam two different things at the same time are perfect; just the right size for a single meal and very energy efficient; a good investment.

# SMOKED MACKEREL WITH CURLY KALE

Smoked mackerel has such a distinctive (and delicious) flavour of its own that it can easily overpower anything you serve with it. However, the cabbage is able to hold its own. This is also a dead simple dish to cook. | Serves 1 (double quantities for 2)

---

1 medium or 2 small parsnips, scrubbed and sliced thickly

1 tbsp olive oil

1 medium onion, peeled and sliced thickly

150g/6oz curly kale, shredded with all coarse stems removed

1 heaped tsp dried sea vegetables/Japanese seaweed

1 small smoked mackerel fillet (peppered or not as you prefer), skinned and broken into large pieces

3-4 tbsp water, water and white wine, or fish stock

sea salt and freshly ground black pepper

½ lemon

---

Steam the sliced parsnips for 8-10 minutes or until they are nearly cooked.

Meanwhile, heat the oil in a saucepan big enough to hold all the vegetables and gently fry the onion for 4-5 minutes or until it is starting to soften. Add kale, the sea vegetables and the par-cooked parsnips and mix gently.

Place the fish over the top, season lightly and add the liquid.

Cover the pan and cook over a low heat for approximately 15 minutes or until the kale is cooked.

Serve from the pan with a squeeze of lemon.

> Seaweeds, sea vegetables or seaweed condiments work particularly well with strong flavours such as smoked mackerel. They also have the virtue of being extremely nutritious (one of the best sources of iodine) as well as tasty – much better than just using salt.

# MACKEREL BAKED WITH APPLE

Mackerel are such a rich fish that they really benefit from the acidity of the sharp apples. This dish works really well with a baked potato to soak up the delicious juices and a green vegetable. | Serves 1 (double quantities for 2)

---

1 tbsp olive oil

1 small onion, finely sliced

¼ small-medium Bramley cooking apple or 1 small, tart eating apple, peeled and sliced

1 sprig fresh rosemary or ½ tsp dried rosemary

1 small mackerel, filleted or not as you feel inclined

4 tbsp dry white wine

sea salt or seaweed condiment and freshly ground black pepper

---

Heat the oil in a pan big enough to take the mackerel. Add the onions and apples, cover the pan and cook them gently for 15 minutes or till they are quite soft. Add the rosemary and season lightly with the sea salt or seaweed condiment.

Lay the mackerel on top of the onion mixture, pour around the wine, re-cover and continue to cook gently for a further 15-20 minutes or till the fish is cooked.

Serve at once with the baked potato and a green vegetable.

*Baking potatoes, for those living on their own, always seems a terrible waste of oven energy. Although I rarely use a microwave for cooking, this does seem the one occasion where a dual operation microwave comes into its own. You can speed up the cooking time (using the microwave on low or medium) but still get a nice crispy skin by using the dual fan oven function at 180 or 190 degrees.*

# STIR FRIED TUNA WITH MANGETOUT

Stir fries are great if you are only cooking for one or two as they are very energy efficient (most of the work going into preparation rather than cooking) and quick to prepare – not to mention tasty, nutritious and low fat…

This is quite a substantial meal but if you feel you need it, accompany it with 75g/3oz boiled wholemeal rice but do not forget that this will take a lot longer to cook than your stir fry. Alternatively, use quinoa. | Serves 1 (double quantities for 2)

---

2 anchovies and 1 tbsp oil from the anchovy tin
2 cloves garlic, peeled and halved if they are very large
½ small red chilli, deseeded and sliced thinly
15g/½oz ginger root, peeled and cut into thin matchsticks
100g/4oz choi sum, pak choi or other Chinese greens, washed and dried and chopped roughly
50g/2oz mangetout, trimmed and halved
3 spring onions, chopped roughly
1 small tuna steak, cut in quite large dice
juice ½ lime
soya sauce

---

Heat the oil in a wok or wide frying pan. Add the anchovies, garlic, chillies and ginger and fry briskly, without burning, for 3-5 minutes.

Chop whatever greens you are using roughly and add to the mix.

Cover and cook for 3 minutes or until the greens are well wilted but not overcooked.

Add the mangetout and continue to cook, covered, for another 2 minutes. You want them to soften slightly but still be crunchy.

Add the tuna chunks, increase the heat and continue to cook uncovered, stirring continually so that all sides of the tuna chunks come into contact with the pan. Depending on how rare you like your tuna, cook for between 1 and 3 minutes.

Season to taste with the lime juice and soya sauce. Serve at once.

> Rice is not, on the whole, a good grain for diabetics, especially white rice which tends to be pretty high on the Glycaemic Index (50-70). However, wholemeal brown rice (with husks still on) is much better, hardly surprisingly, coming in the mid 20s on Glycaemic Load tables. Since curry does seem to demand a rice accompaniment, go for wholegrain of brown rather than white.

# SMOKED HADDOCK PIE

A pie with a bit of a difference as the potatoes are at the bottom rather than the top. If you are on your own, it will reheat well for a second meal. | Serves 2

---

3 medium potatoes, well scrubbed

2 tbsp olive oil

2 medium leeks, cleaned and sliced thickly

2 medium courgettes, wiped and thickly sliced

1½ heaped tsp dried oregano

400g tin chopped tomatoes

2 fillets smoked haddock (undyed), skinned

sea salt and freshly ground black pepper

1 tbsp mixed pumpkin and sunflower seeds or ½ small pack plain potato crisps

---

Slice the potatoes thickly and steam until cooked.

Heat the oven to 180C/350F/Gas mark 4.

Meanwhile, heat the oil in a wide pan and add the leeks. Cook gently for 5 minutes then add the courgettes and the oregano and continue to cook a little more briskly for a further 5-10 minutes or until both leeks and courgettes are lightly browned. Add the tomatoes and continue to cook for another few minutes until the vegetables are well amalgamated.

Lay the potato slices out in the bottom of a pie dish. Lay the smoked haddock fillets out on top of the potatoes and season well.

Spoon the vegetables over the fish. Cover the dish with a lid or foil and bake for 30 minutes.

Remove from the oven, top with the seeds or crisps, run under a hot grill for a couple of minutes to brown them and serve with a green vegetable.

*Always avoid any smoked haddock which looks bright orange/yellow as you can be almost sure that it has been dyed, not smoked! Real smoked haddock should be a pale luminous yellow – the white flesh of the fish just coloured by the peat, oak and silver birch over which they were smoked.*

# POACHED TROUT WITH RHUBARB SAUCE

Rhubarb is seriously delicious with fish but it is only available for a relatively short time each year. But the same principle can be applied with other tart fruits such as gooseberry, kiwi, or apple, all of which go well with a relatively rich fish such as a trout.

Serve with mashed potato or sweet potato and a green vegetable. | Serves 1 (double quantities for 2)

---

1 rainbow trout, cleaned and with its head removed or not as you like

2 slices lemon + ½ lemon

6 tbsp white wine or water

50g/2oz fresh rhubarb (chopped), or gooseberries (topped and tailed), or kiwi fruits (peeled and sliced) or tart apples (peeled, cored and sliced)

15g/½ oz butter

4 tbsp cream, normal cow's milk, oat cream or soya cream

salt, white pepper

a little caster sugar (optional)

---

Put the trout in a lidded pan big enough to hold it with the lemon slices and the wine or water.

Cover it and cook it gently (8-10) minutes or until the fish lifts easily off the bone.

Meanwhile chop the rhubarb or other fruit and stew it gently with the butter in a pan. When it is cooked, pureé it in a food processor and add the cream, seasoning and lemon juice to taste. If the sauce is too thick (it should be the consistency of double cream) add a little of the juices from cooking the fish. If it is too tart, add a pinch of sugar to take the edge off the sharpness.

To serve, remove the fish from the pan, skin and fillet it, lay on a plate and spoon over the sauce.

> Diabetics who are concerned about their fat intake might rather use a soya or an oat cream than regular cow's milk cream. Both are low fat and actually taste remarkably good, especially in a dish like this when you really would not realise you were not eating 'real' cream. Both are available in some supermarkets and in most health food stores.

# FILLET OF COD WITH CHILLI

This is a very simple dish but looks – and tastes – really good. The fieriness of the chillies goes well with the 'cool' flavour of the fish – but you need to be careful not to overdo them. | Serves 1 (double quantities for 2)

---

1 tbsp olive oil

1 small leek

½ head fennel

1 scant tsp dried dill or 2 tsp fresh dill

½ small red chilli – more if you want it hotter

5 cherry tomatoes, quartered

1 piece cod fillet (approx 100g/4oz)

2 tbsp white wine

sea salt (or seaweed condiment) and freshly ground black pepper

¼ lemon

---

Heat the oil in a smallish pan.

Slice the leek and fennel finely and add to the pan along with the dill.

Cut the chilli open and remove the seeds and pith – slice into very thin slivers and add to the vegetables.

Cook, uncovered, for 7-8 minutes or until the fennel is starting to soften.

Add the tomatoes, cover and cook gently for another 15 minutes.

Lay the cod fillet on top of the vegetables and sprinkle with salt and seaweed condiment and freshly ground black pepper.

Pour the wine around the sides.

Cover and cook gently for a further 5-7 minutes or until the fish is cooked.

Serve with a wedge of lemon and a green vegetable such as green beans or spinach.

> Because cod is one of the most over-fished and threatened of fish species be careful what you buy. Only buy fish that have good sustainable credentials, the most reliable being that of the Marine Stewardship Council. Look for an oval blue badge with Marine Stewardship Council on it.

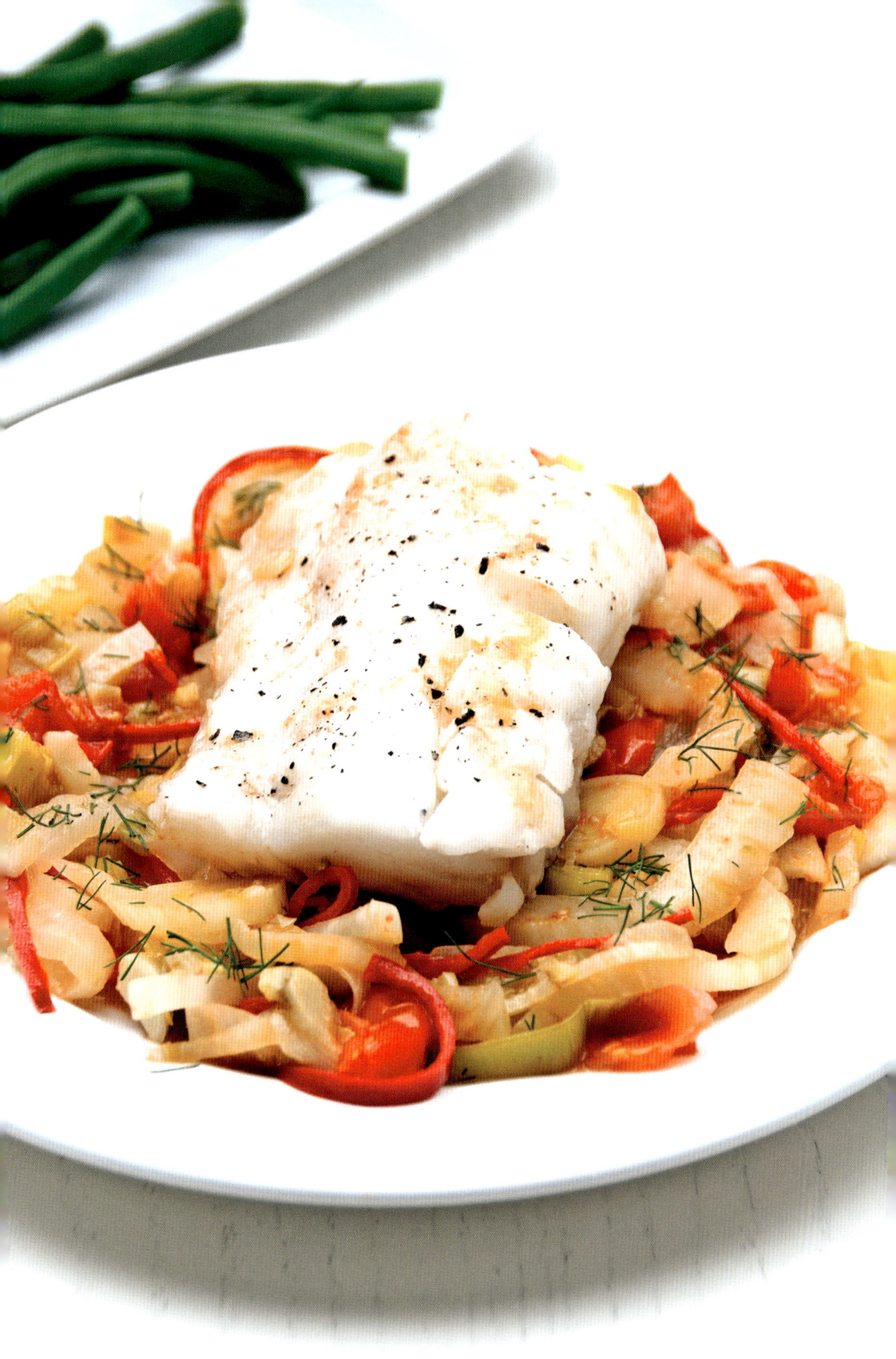

# PEPPER, PEAR AND ANCHOVY SALAD

Delicious cool and refreshing salad for a hot summer day. | Serves 1 (double quantities for 2)

---

1 level tbsp good mayonnaise – homemade or good quality 'bought'

1-2 anchovy fillets, chopped small

salt, pepper and lemon juice

½ medium red pepper, deseeded and finely sliced

½ fresh pear, peeled and sliced thinly – save the other half to have with a slice of blue cheese for dessert...

several leaves of a crispy lettuce such as iceberg or cos

---

Put the mayonnaise in a bowl, add the anchovy.

Mix well and then season to taste with salt, pepper and lemon juice but take care not to over salt as the saltiness of the anchovies will develop in the mayonnaise. The mayonnaise should be of a 'light coating consistency' – like double cream; if it is too thick, thin it with a little boiling water.

Add the peppers and pears and toss gently till both fruit and vegetable are well coated with the dressing.

Serve on a bed of crisp iceberg lettuce.

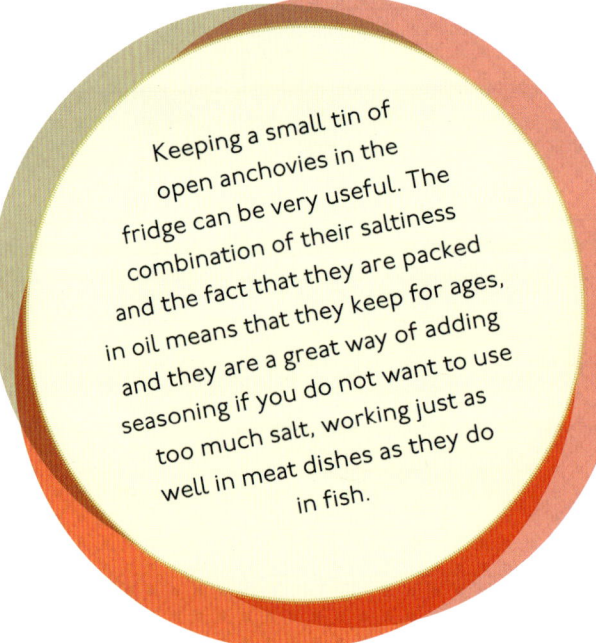

Keeping a small tin of open anchovies in the fridge can be very useful. The combination of their saltiness and the fact that they are packed in oil means that they keep for ages, and they are a great way of adding seasoning if you do not want to use too much salt, working just as well in meat dishes as they do in fish.

# BEEF

SLOW COOK POT ROAST
BEEF CASSEROLE WITH BUTTERNUT SQUASH
BOBOTIE
OXTAIL STEW
MINCED BEEF WITH CURLY KALE
STEAK WITH GARLIC

# SLOW COOK POT ROAST

One of the problems with cooking small joints of meat is that they dry out very quickly – but if you pot roast them, this doesn't happen. However, the meat will certainly benefit from long slow cooking and from being left overnight as the recipe suggests.

If the joint is still slightly larger than you need for one meal, the leftovers will make really delicious cold beef for a salad or sandwiches, layered with horseradish. Meanwhile, the extra juices will give you one or two bowls of mouth-watering beef broth. | Serves 2

---

small topside of beef – approx 750g/1½ lbs

4 small onions, peeled but left whole

4 cloves garlic, peeled but left whole

4 button mushrooms

2 medium carrots, scrubbed and halved

4 bay leaves

1 level tsp black peppercorns

1 glass red wine

50g/2oz black olives

---

Put the meat in a heavy lidded casserole which holds it fairly snugly.

Surround it with the onions, mushrooms and carrots, add the bay leaves, black peppercorns and the wine then add water until the meat is covered. Cover the casserole and cook in a low oven (150C/300F/Gas mark 2) or over a very low heat for 2-4 hours. You could also cook it in a slow cooker overnight.

Allow the meat to cool in the juices, then chill until any fat solidifies on top. Remove the fat and gently reheat the casserole. Add the olives and adjust the seasoning of the juices to taste. Serve with baked potatoes and a green vegetable.

> Most people assume that for a casserole to taste good you need first of all to fry the vegetables and, indeed, the meat but this is not necessarily true. You get a different flavour, if you do not fry, but some people would think it was a 'cleaner' flavour. One of the best beef dishes I ever had was a Victorian 'beef stew' which just required you to cook a joint of beef with some seasoning, just covered in water, very, very, very slowly.

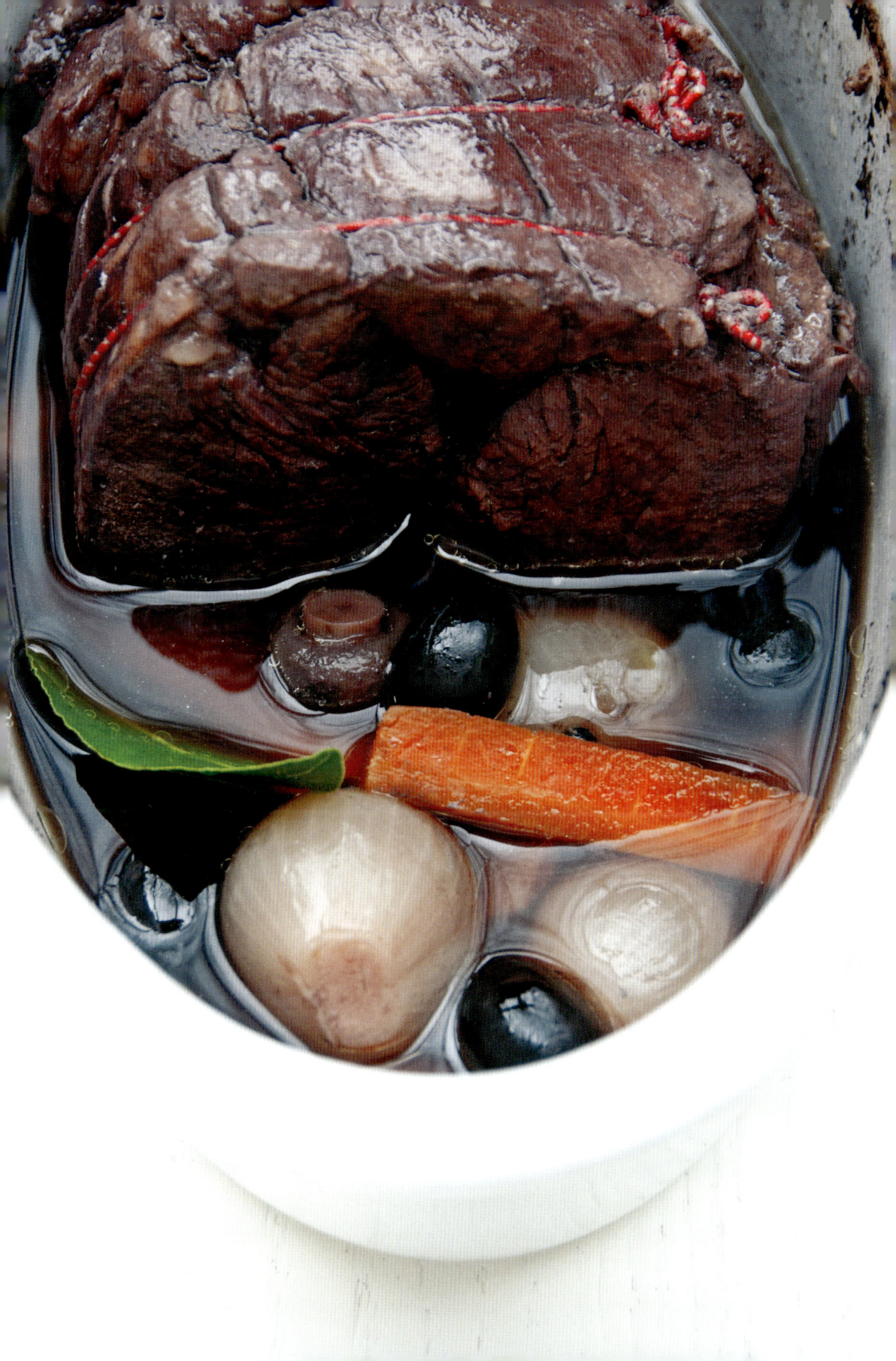

# BEEF CASSEROLE WITH BUTTERNUT SQUASH

Being a lazy cook, I really like all-in-one dishes where at least one vegetable is incorporated. This one is a great winter dish – it not only tastes warming but looks it too. You can use a cheaper cut of beef if you want, but if so, increase the cooking time to 1½ - 2 hours.

The Marsala will give a slightly richer, sweeter flavour than a normal red wine.

This casserole will benefit from being cooked in advance as it allows time for the flavours to mature. It also freezes well so, if you want to double up on the quantities, you could freeze half for a future occasion. | Serves 2

---

2 tablespoons olive oil

small knob (approx 25g/1oz) fresh ginger root, peeled and cut into thin matchsticks

100g/4oz shallots or very small onions, peeled

1 small butternut squash, peeled, deseeded and cut into medium-size cubes

1 level dessertspoon flour

sea salt and freshly ground black pepper

250g/9oz braising beef, trimmed and diced

120ml/4floz red wine or Marsala

150ml/¼ pint water

2 bay leaves

---

Heat the oil in a small but heavy casserole. Add the ginger and shallots or onions and fry gently for several minutes.

Add the squash and continue to fry fairly briskly until both are lightly tanned. Meanwhile, season the flour generously and toss the diced beef in it.

Add the beef to the pot and continue to cook briskly for 3-4 minutes or until the beef and flour are well browned.

Add the wine or Marsala and use a wooden spoon to deglaze and remove the stuck bits of flour from the bottom of the pan. Then add the water and bay leaves and mix well.

Bring slowly to the boil, stirring continuously until the sauce thickens somewhat. Lower the heat to a gentle simmer and cook for 45 minutes to 1 hour or until the beef is tender and the squash very soft. Adjust the seasoning to taste and serve with a fresh green vegetable.

> Not that long ago fresh ginger root was an exotic luxury but these days it is available in most supermarkets. However, if you cannot find any, substitute 1 heaped teaspoon dried ginger.

# BOBOTIE

Bobotie is the traditional dish of South Africa and comes out a bit like a spicy moussaka although with a more interesting blend of flavours. Surprisingly, if you have any over, or if you are on your own, it also tastes jolly good cold. | Serves 2

---

1 slice thick wholemeal bread

300 ml/½ pint milk

225g/8oz minced beef

1 tbsp olive oil

1 medium onion, finely chopped

1 tbsp curry powder – mild or strong depending on how hot your want your Bobotie

juice 2 small lemons

½ tsp dark brown sugar

salt and pepper

2 small eggs

25g/1oz toasted nibbed almonds or broken cashews

25g/1oz raisins

---

Heat the oven to 180C/350F/Gas mark 4.

Soak the bread in half the milk for a couple of minutes, then mince it roughly with the beef in a food processor.

Heat the oil in a pan and lightly fry the onions with the curry powder.

Mix the lemon juice, sugar, salt, pepper and 1 egg in a bowl.

Add the onion mixture, then the bread and meat and mix them all well together. Spoon them into an ovenproof dish.

Mix the remaining egg and milk with the almonds and raisins, season it liberally and pour it over the meat mixture, allowing the liquid to soak well in and making sure that the fruit and nuts are well spread over the top.

Bake, uncovered, for 30 minutes or till the top is lightly browned and puffed.

Serve with boiled rice or quinoa (if you do not do so well with rice), homemade chutney and a green salad.

> As diabetics will know, white rice is relatively high on the Glycaemic Index and can send some (but not all) diabetics' blood sugars soaring. Wholegrain rice has less of an instant hit (because you have to digest the whole grain rather than just the starchy insides) but has a quite different, much nuttier texture. Some people may prefer to use quinoa, the highly nutritious South American grain which cooks up very easily and is a good rice substitute in most dishes.

# OXTAIL STEW

This is a real classic – and so easy to cook. If you can get big pieces of oxtail you will also get the benefit of the amazingly nutritious and delicious marrow to be found in the middle of the bone. However, you will probably need to buy your oxtail from a butcher as few supermarkets will stock it.

You need to make the stew 24 hours in advance so that the flavours will have a chance to develop overnight and the fat will rise to the top so that you can remove it – important for those who are trying to keep the fat intake down. But even when you have removed the fat, the stew will still have a delicious, slightly unctuous texture. | Serves 2

1 tbsp olive oil
1 medium onion, peeled and finely chopped
1 stick celery, finely chopped
1 rasher fatty bacon, finely chopped
4 large pieces oxtail
1 tbsp well seasoned flour
400ml/14floz beef or vegetable stock
2 bay leaves
2 sprigs parsley, chopped

In a heavy pan heat the oil and add the onion, celery and bacon. Fry gently for 10-15 minutes or until the vegetables are lightly browned.

Toss the oxtail in the seasoned flour then increase the heat under the pan and add the oxtail pieces. Fry briskly till lightly browned, add the rest of the flour, stir well around then gradually add the stock, stirring well so you get all the burnt bits off the bottom of the pan.

Add the bay leaves, bring slowly to the boil, then reduce the heat, cover the pan and simmer very gently for 1½-2 hours. The meat should be falling off the bone.

Adjust the seasoning to taste, sprinkled with the parsley, and serve with baked potatoes and a green vegetable.

> Many classic dishes tend to get ignored by those on 'special diets' but they really should not be. Most are free of all the fat, sugar and salt which are so over-represented in many pre-prepared foods – and are so bad for all of us, but especially for diabetics. What is more, properly cooked, most of them taste just great.

# MINCED BEEF WITH CURLY KALE

A lovely rich and spicy all-in-one-pot meal. Yet another dish that benefits from being cooked in advance and left overnight for its flavours to 'mature'. There are so many vegetables already in the dish that you should not need any extras. | Serves 2

---

1 tbsp olive oil
1 red onion, peeled and chopped
1 clove garlic, peeled and sliced
1 medium carrot, scrubbed and sliced in rings
½ medium red pepper, cut in large dice
1 small hot green chilli, deseeded and chopped very small
75g/3oz small button mushrooms, wiped and halved
100g/4oz piece celeriac, peeled and cut in largish dice
1 tsp dried thyme
175g/6oz minced beef
400g tin chopped tomatoes
2 tbsp red wine
sea salt and freshly ground black pepper
½ x 400g tin aduki beans
100g/4oz curly kale, washed, its stalks removed and chopped

---

Heat the oil in a large pan and add the onion and garlic. Cook gently for a few minutes then add the carrot, pepper, chilli and mushrooms. Continue to cook for a further couple of minutes without burning.

Add the celeriac, thyme and the beef. Again, stir well and continue to cook for a further few minutes.

Finally, add the tomatoes, wine and some seasoning. Bring to the boil, cover, reduce the heat and simmer gently for 40 minutes.

Add the aduki beans and the kale, mix well and cook for a further 10 minutes or until the kale is cooked.

Curly kale is a bit of an acquired taste as it is quite strong – although it is 'tamed' by the many other strong flavours in this dish. However, bear in mind that it is strongly anti-inflammatory, very low Glycaemic Load (a mere 3…), very high in vitamins A, C and K and a reasonable source of manganese, potassium and copper.

# STEAK WITH GARLIC

If you are on your own and fancy a treat – this is it! It is incredibly simple but will improve even the best cut of steak.

---

1 steak per person, cut of your choice
sea salt and freshly ground
black pepper
4 cloves of garlic per person

---

Lay the steak out on a plate and grate over a little sea salt and black pepper. Crush 2 cloves of garlic in a garlic press and spread over the steak.

Turn the steak and repeat the process on the other side. Leave for 1-2 hours to absorb the flavours.

Grill, barbecue or fry to your taste and serve with baked potatoes and a green vegetable or salad. Or, if you don't want to heat an oven for just one baked potato, put your steak on a thick slice of really nice wholemeal bread which will absorb its juices so that they don't get wasted and serve with a green vegetable.

## Steaks

You can go either for maximum flavour, which may involve a bit of chewing, or maximum tenderness, which may mean a rather more delicate flavour.

**Fillet, chateaubriand, mignon or tournedos** – all cut from the fillet, the lean and boneless part of the animal which lies just below the ribs: the tenderest and most expensive; very lean so can benefit from larding with fat.

**Porterhouse, T-bone, sirloin, entrecote** – larger cuts of steak which come from the rib and back of the animal – lots of flavour, more fat but not as tender.

**Rump** – a larger joint from the hind leg – lots of flavour but not so tender.

Take your pick.

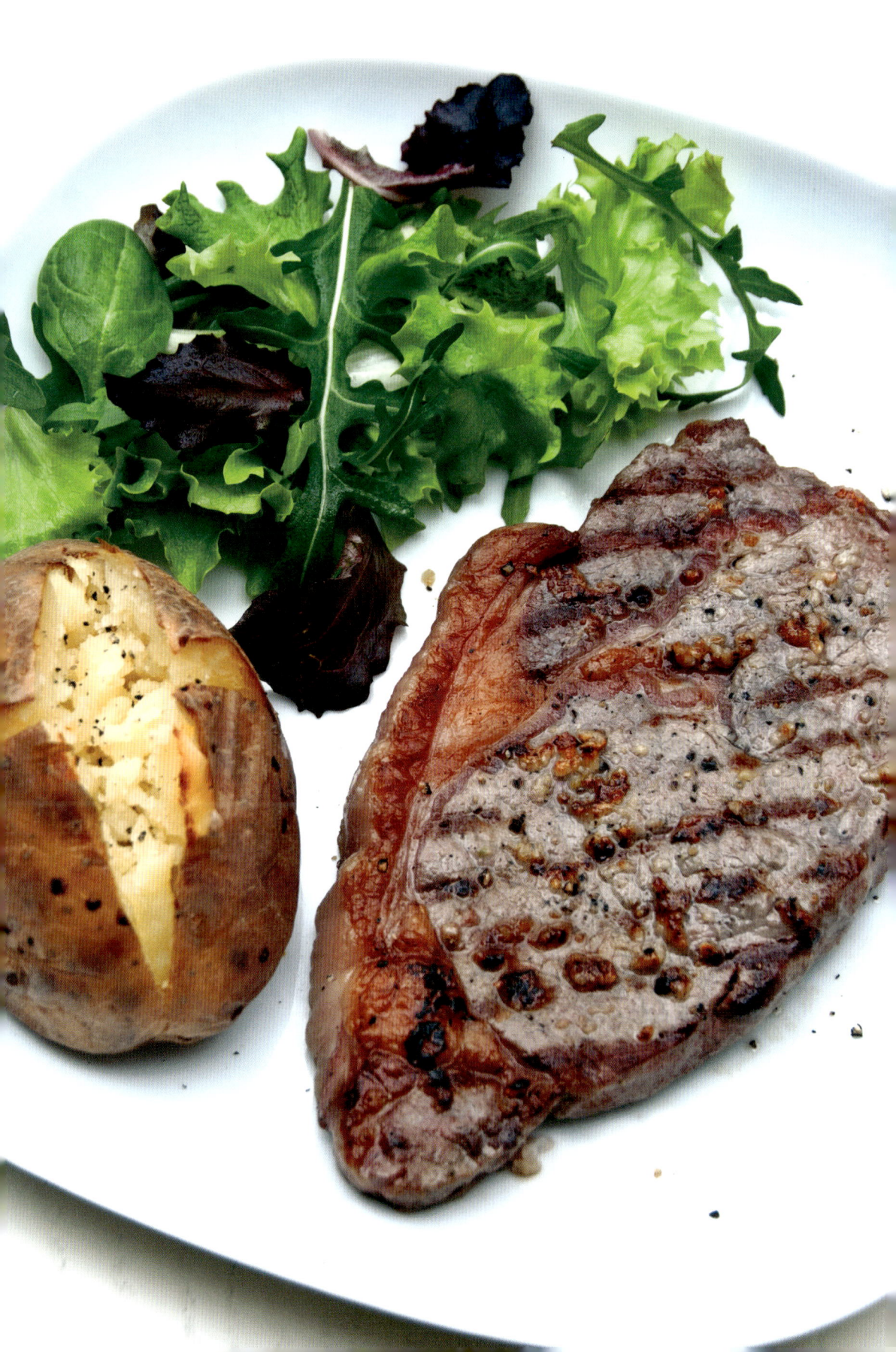

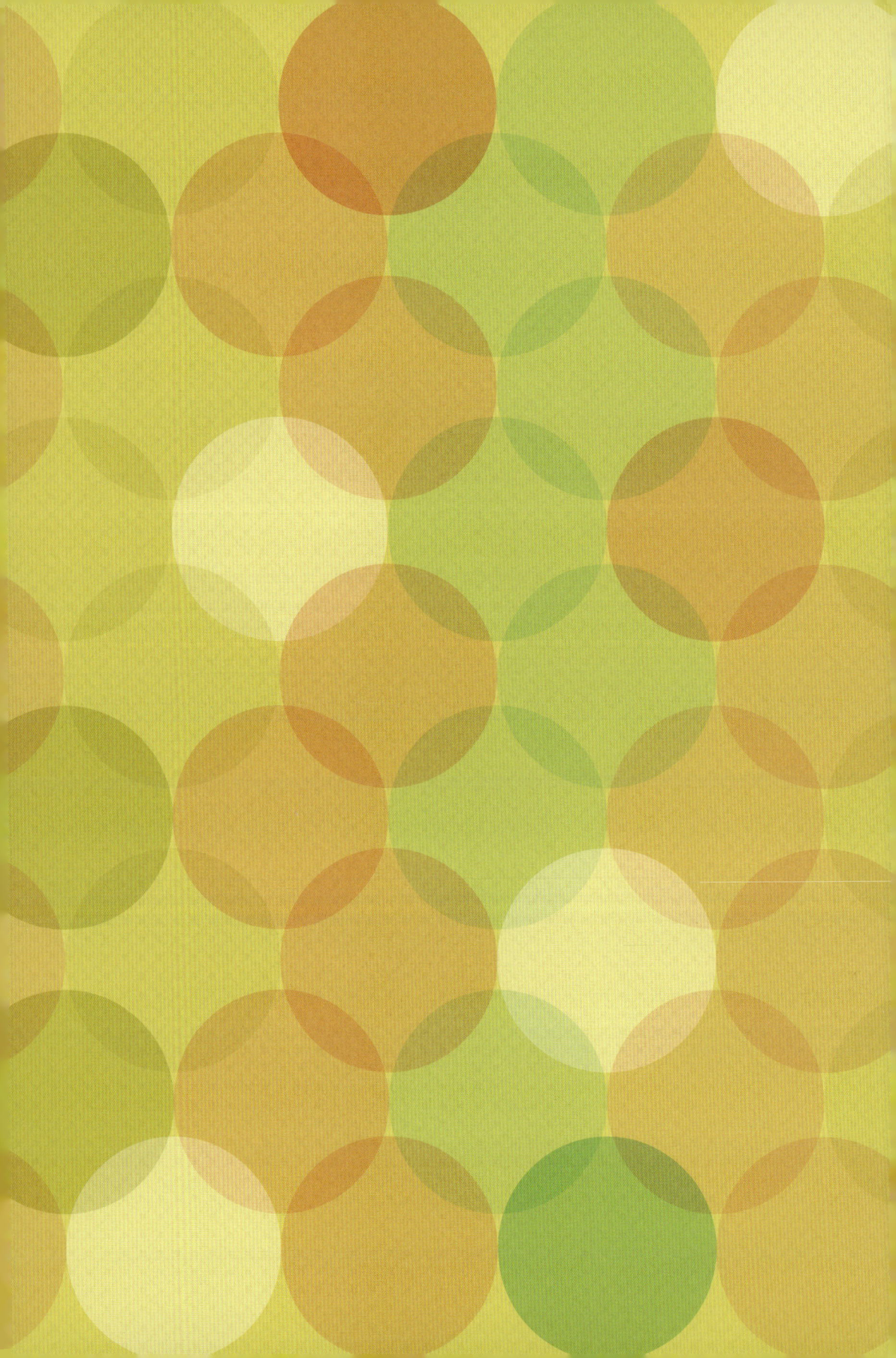

# LAMB

LAMB TAJINE
LAMB'S KIDNEYS WITH CHESTNUTS AND MARSALA
OYSTER-STUFFED HALF SHOULDER OF LAMB
LAMB AND PEPPER KEBABS FOR THE BARBECUE
RACK OF LAMB WITH MUSTARD CRUST

# LAMB TAJINE

A tajine is a slow-cook North African stew, originally cooked over an open fire in one of those wonderful tall-lidded earthenware pots. Because of the complex mix of flavours it really benefits from the long slow cooking and is often better on day two than day one – so don't worry if you seem to have more than you need. | Serves 2

---

2 tbsp olive oil

2 heaped tsp ground cumin

1 level tsp ground coriander

1-2 large cloves garlic, peeled and sliced

1 small onion, peeled and sliced fairly thinly

1 small-medium carrot, scrubbed and cut into thin rounds

1 stick celery, chopped small

350g/12oz lamb neck fillet, cut in thick slices

½ medium aubergine (eggplant), halved lengthways and sliced

2 dried limes (you can buy them in any Middle Eastern shop)

rind of ¼ lemon

200g/7oz fresh (chopped) or tinned chopped tomatoes

180ml/6floz vegetable stock

50g/2oz fresh spinach (proper spinach rather than baby leaves if you can find it), chopped roughly

250g/9oz cooked chickpeas – you can use tinned

sea salt and freshly ground black pepper

1-2 handfuls of fresh coriander

harissa sauce

---

Heat the oil in a heavy pan – a cast iron one is ideal – and add the ground cumin and coriander, garlic, onion, carrot and celery. Fry fairly briskly without burning for 4-5 minutes or until all the vegetables are starting to soften slightly.

Add the lamb and continue to cook fairly briskly for another few minutes.

Add the aubergine, stir well around, then add the limes, lemon rind, tomatoes and stock. Bring to the boil then cover and reduce the heat to a bare simmer.

Cook for 1½ hours over a very low heat – the surface of the stew should be scarcely moving.

Add the chickpeas and spinach and some seasoning, bring back to the simmer and cook for another 45 minutes.

Harissa is the classic North African condiment found on every table in Tunisia and Algeria and on most in Morocco. Although there are as many recipes as there are families who make it, the main ingredients are hot chilli peppers and olive oil and can also include cumin, red peppers, garlic, coriander and lemon juice and in some areas can taste quite smoky. It is used not only as a condiment but as an ingredient in stews and to rub into and flavour meat or aubergines.

It is worth buying a good quality harissa as the flavour will be more complex and interesting rather than just hot – and it will last a long time. However, it does come in small pots and can be used in all kinds of non-African dishes such as on pasta or pizza or even in sandwiches.

When you are ready serve, adjust the seasoning to taste and add the chopped fresh coriander.

You can serve the tajine alone or with pita or flatbread – and, of course, the harissa – start with no more than 1 teaspoon per serving as, depending on which one you buy, it can be quite hot and overpower the lamb.

# LAMB'S KIDNEYS WITH CHESTNUTS AND MARSALA

Kidneys are a perfect meat for those on their own as you can literally buy just one or two. They are also delicious – and nutritious. Particularly in this dish… | Serves 2 (halve quantities if you want to only serve one)

---

2 tbsp olive oil

1 small onion, peeled and very finely chopped

sea salt

50g/2oz chestnut mushrooms, wiped and sliced

50g/2oz cooked chestnuts, sliced thickly (you can buy small tins in most delicatessens)

1 heaped tsp seasoned flour

4 lamb's kidneys, trimmed and halved

150ml/¼ pint miso or vegetable stock

4 tbsp Marsala or heavy red wine

2 slices Parma ham, cut into small squares (you can buy Parma ham by the slice at most deli counters)

freshly ground black pepper

---

Heat the oil in a small heavy pan and add the onion and a small pinch of salt to stop them burning. Cook gently for 5 minutes or until the onion is softening then add the mushrooms and continue to cook for another 3-4 minutes. Add the chestnuts.

Meanwhile, toss the kidneys in the seasoned flour.

Add them to the vegetables, stir well then add the miso or stock and the Marsala. Bring to the simmer and simmer gently for 4-5 minutes or until the kidneys are just cooked.

Add the Parma ham and mix well. Season with black pepper – if you have used the miso you are unlikely to need any extra salt. Serve with boiled rice and a green vegetable or salad.

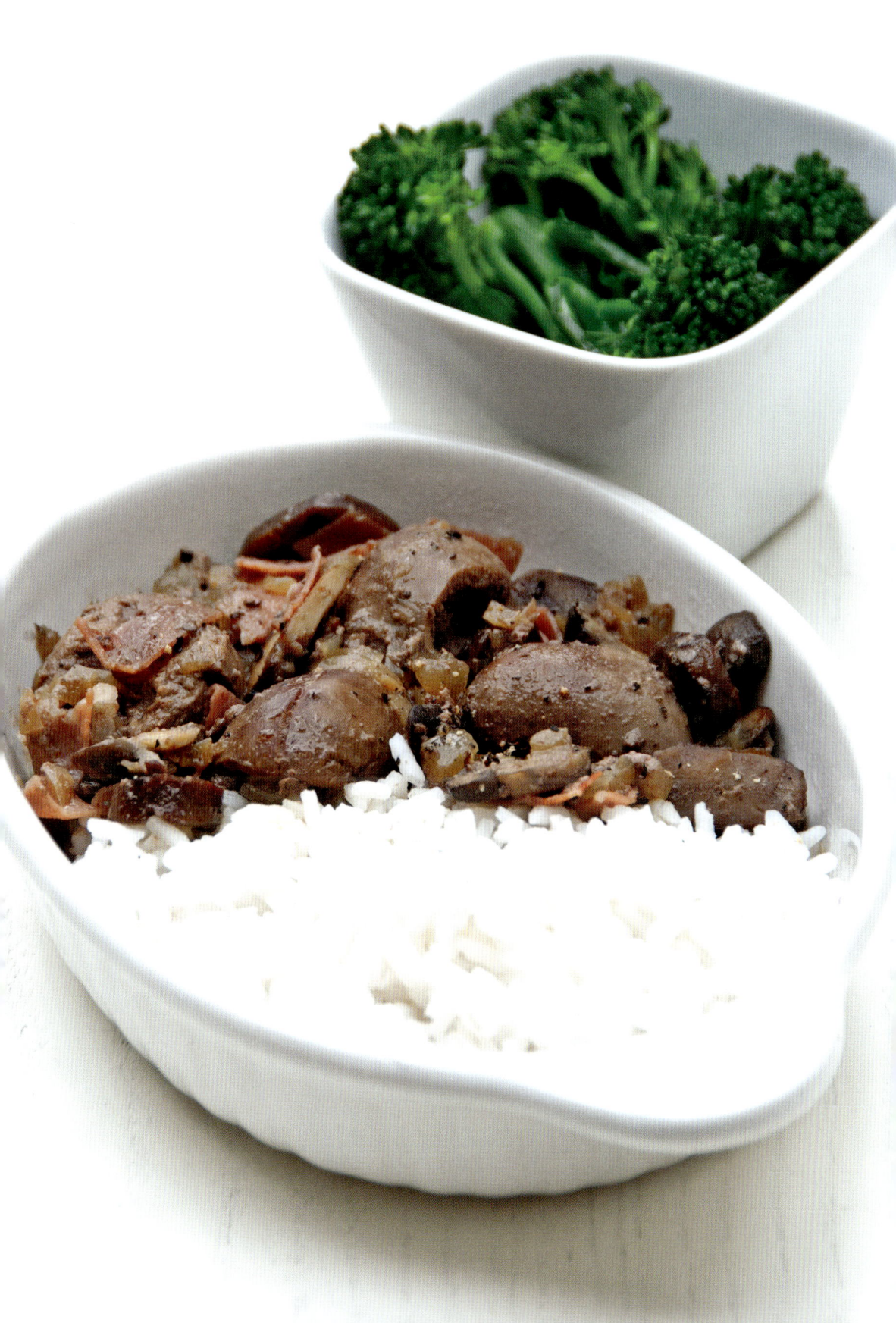

# OYSTER-STUFFED HALF SHOULDER OF LAMB

While a whole shoulder of lamb would be a good deal too much for two people, a small half shoulder would be perfect, just leaving you enough for cold lamb with salad, lamb sandwiches or a dish such as the Bobotie in the beef section, which could also be made with lamb.

Smoked mussels and oysters are available in most supermarkets and are relatively cheap and very tasty. | Serves 2

---

1 tbsp olive oil

50g/2oz field mushrooms, wiped and sliced

½ x 85g tin smoked oysters or mussels – save the rest to use in a salad or sandwich with a little lettuce and a squeeze of lemon juice

2 sprigs of fresh thyme or 1 heaped tsp dried thyme

sea salt and freshly ground black pepper

1 small half shoulder of lamb, boned out but not rolled

---

Heat the oven to 180C/350F/Gas mark 4.

Heat the oil in a pan and briskly fry the mushrooms for 2-3 minutes or until their juices run. Remove and mix with the oysters or mussels, their oil and the leaves from the thyme.

Lay out the lamb, season and then lay the oyster mixture down the middle. Roll the lamb, tie neatly with string and lay on a baking tray. Pour any juices that squeezed out over it.

Season, sprinkle with the remaining thyme leaves, cover lightly with foil and bake for 20 minutes per 450g plus an extra 15 minutes. Remove the foil for the last 30 minutes.

When cooked remove to a serving dish and use the juices with a level tablespoon of flour and 300-400ml/10-14floz water, stock or water and wine mixed to make some gravy.

Serve with vegetables of your choice.

> If you have ever done any sailing you will have no difficulty in tying the slip knots used by most butchers to tie up your shoulder of lamb. If you are not good with knots, you can always use elastic bands. The ones that the postmen scatter with such abandon would be just about the right size for a half shoulder.

# LAMB AND PEPPER KEBABS FOR THE BARBECUE

Kebabs are great for small numbers as you only have to make as many as you need and although it is fun cooking them on a barbecue, they will taste 99% as good if cooked under a grill! | Serves 2

---

1 small clove garlic, crushed
4 spring onions, finely chopped
25g/1oz fresh ginger root, peeled and finely chopped
1 level tsp turmeric
juice of 1 small lemon
1 tbsp plain yogurt, cow, goat, sheep or soya
1 tbsp sesame, nut or olive oil
a good shake soy sauce
200g/7oz lamb fillet, trimmed and cut into reasonable chunks – approximately 3cm/1½ inches square
salt and pepper
1 yellow pepper, cut into largish squares
1 decent-sized courgette, wiped and cut in thick rounds

---

Mix all the garlic, spring onions, ginger root, turmeric, lemon juice, yogurt, oil and soy sauce together in a bowl. Add the lamb and mix well. Cover and set aside to marinade for 4-6 hours or overnight.

When ready to cook, remove the meat from the marinade and thread it onto skewers or kebab sticks alternately with the yellow pepper and courgette rounds. Season lightly.

Cook it under a hot grill or on a charcoal barbecue for 5-7 minutes, basting periodically with the remains of the marinade. The lamb needs to be frizzled on the outside but can be pink within.

Serve the kebabs with pita bread and a fresh, green salad.

*This is a relatively complicated marinade but just marinating your lamb (or chicken, or fish) in some lemon juice, a little sea salt and freshly ground black pepper, some good olive oil and, sometimes, a shake of soy sauce for 30 minutes before you cook it can both give ot a more interesting flavour and prevent it drying out in the cooking.*

# RACK OF LAMB WITH MUSTARD CRUST

A rack of lamb is another joint which is good for a small number of people as you can get as few or as many cutlets on it as you need. However, you must be sure, as it is small, that you do not let it dry out – which is why cooking it over the vegetables is a good idea. | Serves 2

2 tablespoons olive oil

1 leek, sliced thickly

1 rasher bacon, chopped roughly

350g/12oz potatoes, scrubbed and sliced thinly

1 small rack of lamb

2 sprigs each fresh rosemary and fresh thyme or 1 level tsp each dried

2 tbsp fresh brown breadcrumbs

2 heaped tsp Dijon mustard

Heat the oven to 180C/350F/Gas mark 4.

Heat the oil in the bottom of a small, heavy oven-proof casserole large enough to hold the lamb. Briskly fry the leek and the bacon till both are lightly coloured, then add the potatoes and continue to fry gently for 5 minutes.

Lay the sprigs of herbs (or sprinkle the dried herbs) over the vegetables.

Mix the breadcrumbs with the mustard and spread the mustard mixture over the lamb.

Lay the lamb on top of the potatoes, skin side up. Cover the casserole tightly and bake in a moderate oven for 20 minutes or until the lamb is cooked to your liking.

Serve the lamb from the pot with the potatoes and a green vegetable.

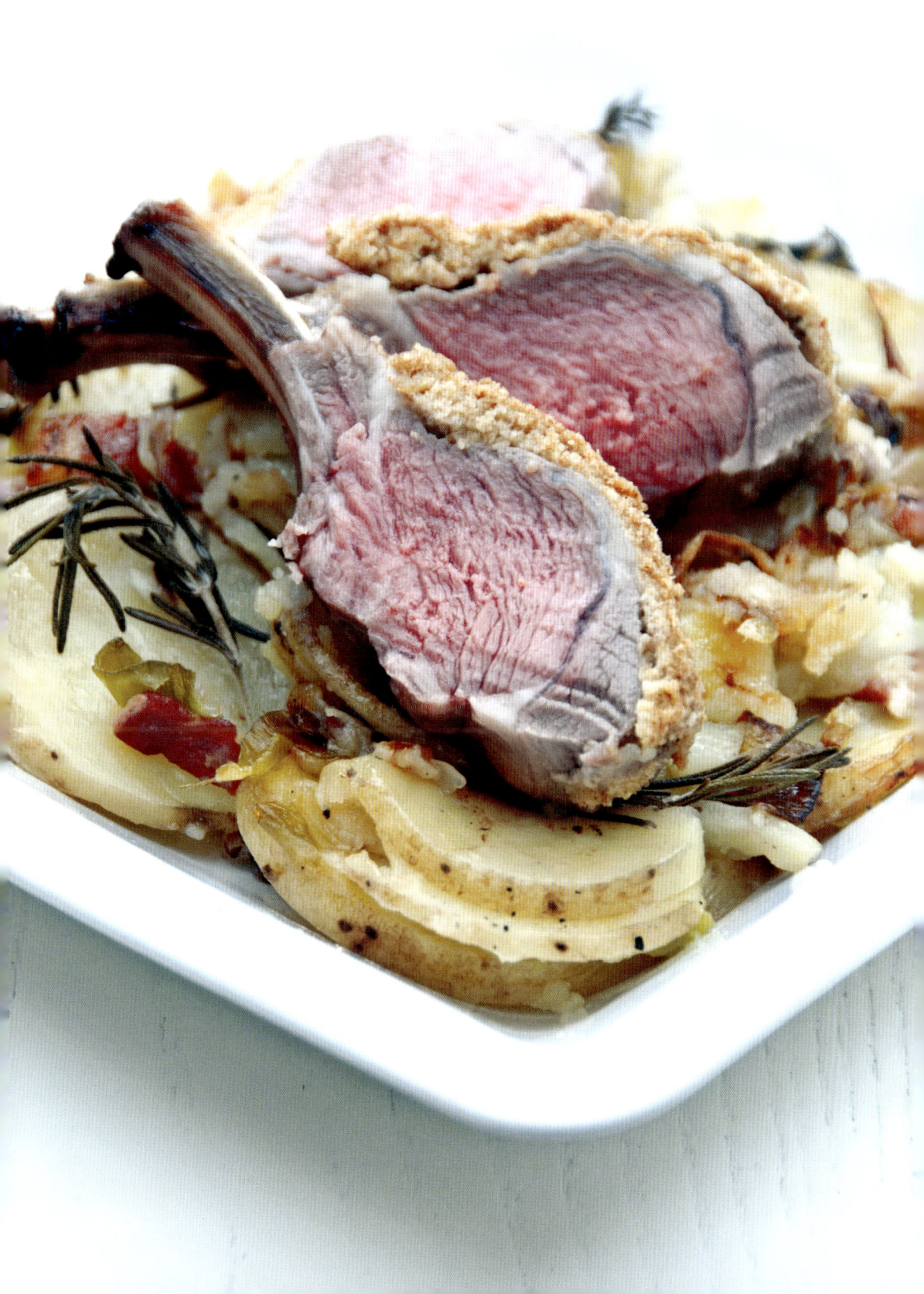

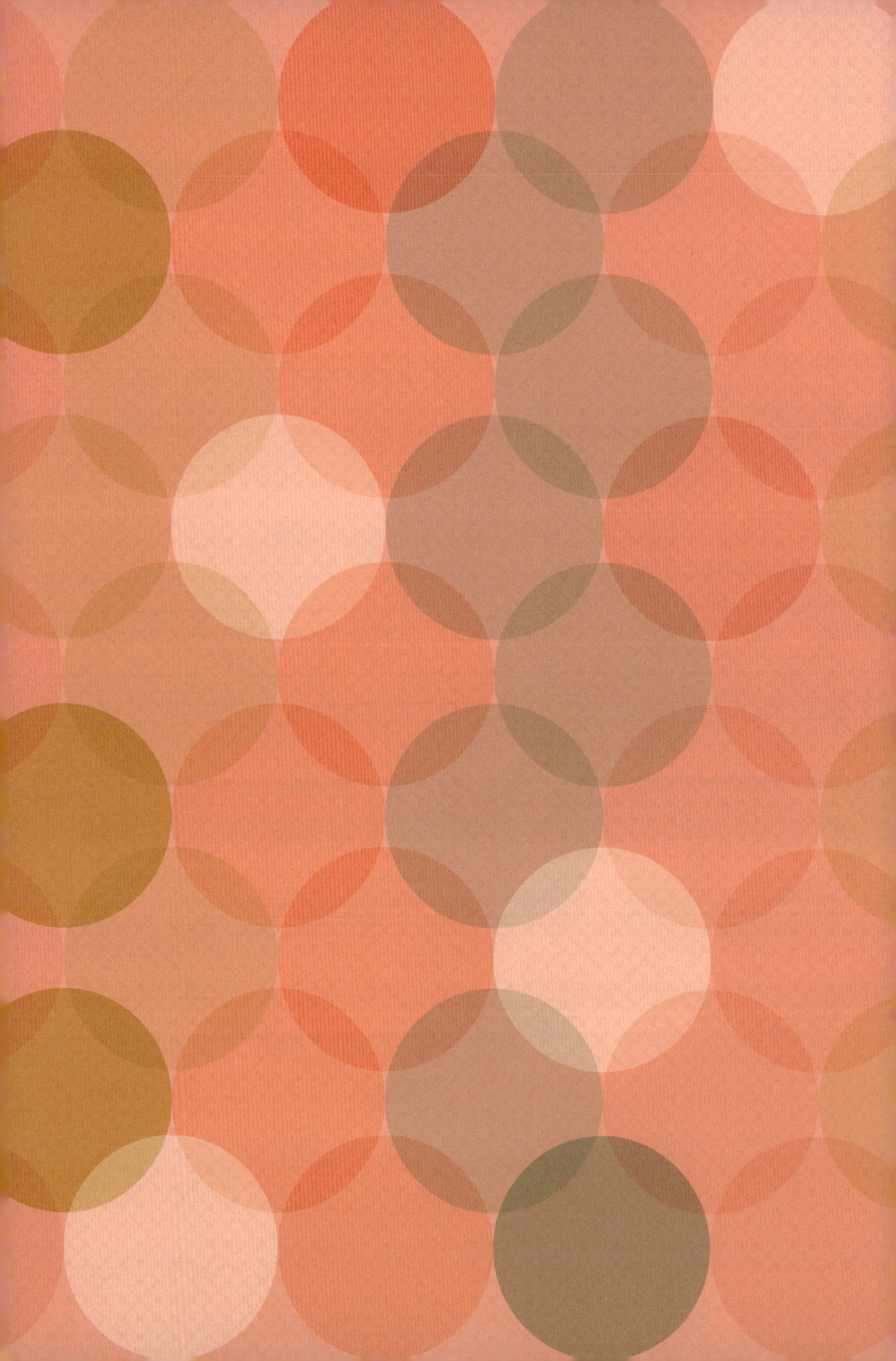

# PORK

SAUSAGE AND BEAN POT
PORK CHOPS WITH APPLE AND ROSEMARY
GAMMON WITH GREEN LENTILS AND CABBAGE
SAUSAGES WITH BEETROOT, BUTTER BEANS
AND HORSERADISH

# SAUSAGE AND BEAN POT

These kinds of bean pots just get better and better the longer you keep them. So if it is more than you need, you can leave the remains in the fridge for two or three days, as long as it is well chilled, so that when you come back to it, it is like a new dish. Just add a little more liquid and away you go. | Serves 2

---

2 tbsp olive oil
2 small red onions, peeled and sliced
2 cloves garlic, peeled and sliced
½ medium leek, trimmed and cut in thick slices
1 stick celery, scrubbed and cut into thick slices
4 button mushrooms, wiped and halved
1 heaped tsp dried mixed herbs
3 tbsp Puy lentils
25g/1oz sun-dried tomatoes, chopped
100g/4oz rough French or Italian sausage, thickly sliced
100ml/4floz red wine
300ml/½ pint vegetable stock
small can (200g) each cannellini and borlotti beans, drained
freshly ground black pepper
1 handful of fresh parsley, roughly chopped

---

Put the oil, onions, garlic, leek, celery, mushrooms and mixed herbs into a heavy flame-proof casserole and fry briskly for 5-10 minutes without burning.

Add the lentils, tomatoes, sausage, red wine and stock. Bring slowly to the boil, cover and simmer for at least an hour.

Add the drained beans and then return to the boil and simmer for a further 15 minutes. If there is too much liquid, continue to cook briskly, with the lid off, for a further five minutes to reduce the juices.

Season with lots of black pepper and salt if you need it – you may not need any if the sausage is very salty.

To serve, reheat and add the parsley just before serving.

Because there are already plenty of vegetables in the bean pot, you may not need any extras, but a fresh green salad afterwards would be good.

> If you cannot get small tins of cannellini and borlotti beans you can use any others – haricot, butterbeans, flageolet, black-eyed pea, kidney etc – but try to use two different ones as it varies the texture and the colour of the bean pot. You could also cook the beans from scratch but that would probably (depending on the bean) involve soaking them overnight first and then boiling them. They will be slightly nicer but you may not wish to go to all that trouble.

# PORK CHOPS WITH APPLE AND ROSEMARY

This is a really delicious way to cook pork – the sharpness of the cooking apple counteracting the richness of the pork. I am giving the ingredients for a single portion but feel free to double up if you want to serve 2 or more. If you are trying to cut down on your fat consumption you will need to trim the fat from the chop and discard it; if you do not eat a lot of fat anyway then you can use it to cook the meat which will give it a better, more intense 'porky' flavour.

| Serves 1

---

1 nice meaty pork chop
1 tbsp olive oil (optional)
½ a small leek, finely sliced
2 shallots, peeled and finely sliced
¼ Bramley cooking apple, cored but not peeled and chopped finely
4 tbsp dry white wine
1 sprig fresh rosemary or ½ tsp dried rosemary
sea salt and coarsely ground black pepper

---

Trim the layer of fat and skin from the outside of the pork chop. If you wish to use the fat to cook the pork, grill the fat and skin until the fat melts and save the liquid fat. Discard the skin.

Pour the liquid fat or the olive oil, if you are using it, into a pan just big enough to hold your chop (or chops) and add the leek, shallots and finely chopped apple.

Cook very gently, covered, for 10-15 minutes or until they are very soft. Add the wine, lay the sprigs of rosemary over the mixture and the pork chop(s) on top.

Grind over a little sea salt and black pepper, cover the pan and cook gently, covered, for 30 minutes or until the pork is cooked through.

Serve with a root vegetable (potatoes, sweet potatoes, celeriac, squash) steamed and mashed and steamed broccoli or green beans.

Bramley apples are the best to use with pork as their acidity counteracts the richness of the pork so well but if you cannot find any, any small sharp eating apple will do instead. If you find yourself with ¾ of a Bramley apple over you can either stew it with a little water and a few raisins (no extra sugar needed) and eat it for breakfast – or mix a few raisins with a few nuts (almonds, walnuts or cashews), pile them in mound in an ovenproof dish, sit the apple over the top, add a little water, cover and bake for 30 minutes and eat as a dessert.

# GAMMON WITH GREEN LENTILS AND CABBAGE

You can buy really small joints of gammon both in the butcher and in supermarkets so it is a perfectly viable joint for one or two people. And of course it keeps very well so the leftovers can be kept in the fridge for a couple of days before you decide to use them in an omelette, a quinoa risotto, a salad or in sandwiches – with a slather of Dijon mustard or horseradish. | Serves 2

---

Approx 450g/1lb piece of gammon, smoked or unsmoked – see below
Approx 350ml/12floz milk – if you wish to keep the fat content low, use an oat or soya milk rather than cow's milk
1 large sprig fresh rosemary or 1 heaped tsp dried
1 tbsp olive oil
1 small onion, peeled and sliced
1 tsp coriander seeds, lightly crushed
sea salt
100g/4oz green lentils
350ml/12floz chicken or vegetable stock
approx ½ a small green cabbage, washed and chopped
freshly ground black pepper

---

Put the gammon in a saucepan just big enough to hold it. Add the rosemary and the milk which should come ⅔ of the way up the meat. Bring to the boil then reduce the heat and simmer, covered for 30-35 minutes.

Meanwhile heat the oil in a deep pan and add the onion and coriander seeds with a pinch of salt. Fry gently for 5-10 minutes, or until they are quite soft. Add the lentils and stock, bring to the boil, cover and simmer for 15 minutes then add the cabbage and mix well.

Transfer the gammon from the saucepan into the one with the lentils and push it down into the lentils.

Cover the dish and continue to cook gently for a further 15-20 minutes or until the cabbage and lentils are both quite cooked.

Adjust the seasoning to taste and serve at once. You should not need any other vegetables.

All bacons and gammons are cured for around 4 days in brine and then 'matured' for a further 7-10 days. However, not all are smoked. Unsmoked bacon and gammon, also known as 'green', is pale pink and has a relatively delicate flavour and does not have very good keeping qualities. Smoked bacon and ham is further dried and smoked, is a darker pink in colour, has a stronger flavour and keeps much better. Which you prefer is a matter of personal taste. While gammon and bacon used to be thought of as very fatty meats (and many people believe that the flavour actually comes from the fat) modern farming methods have produced pork which is relatively low in fat so even if you are on a low-fat diet, it should be OK for you.

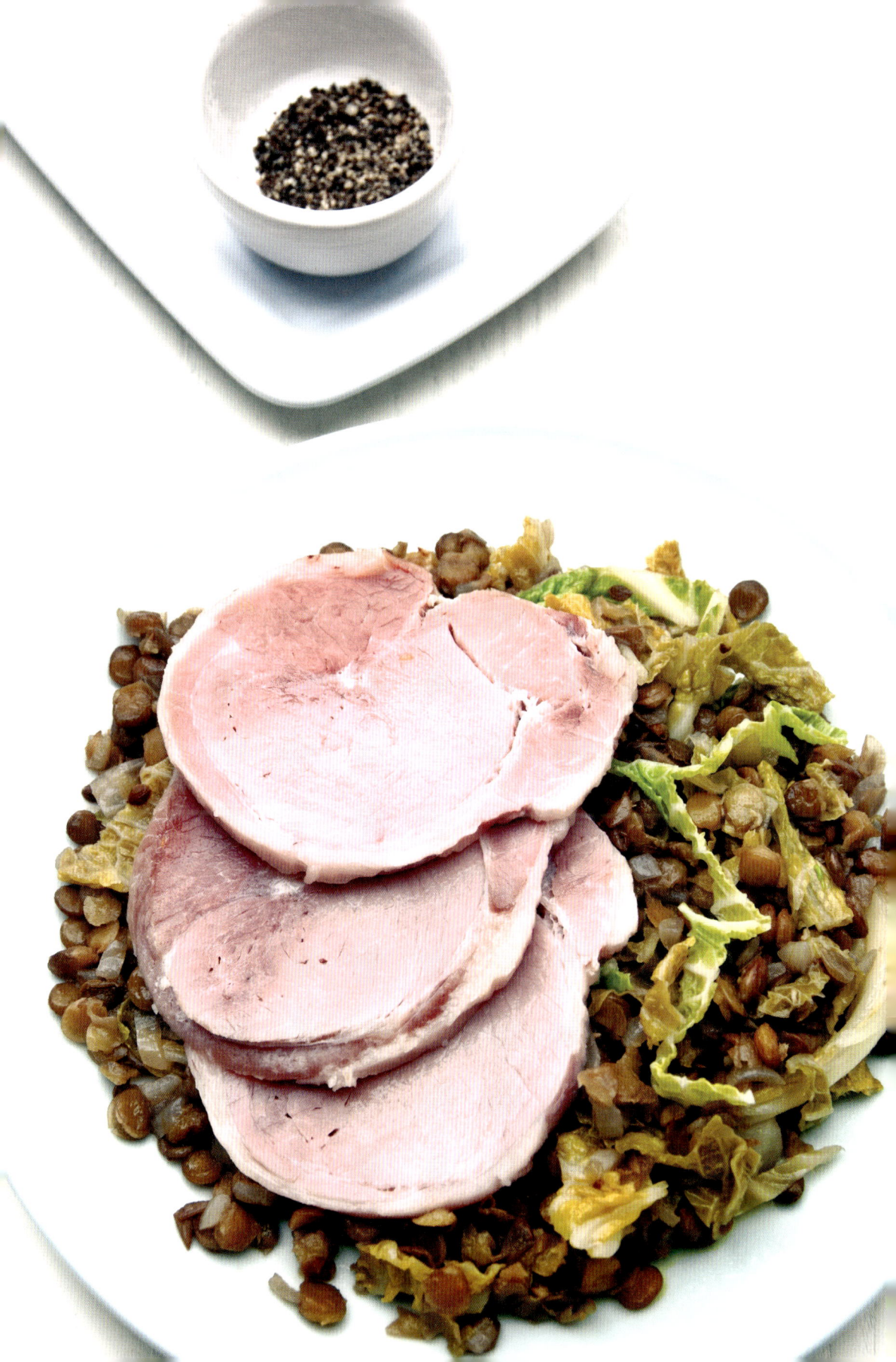

# SAUSAGES WITH BEETROOT, BUTTER BEANS AND HORSERADISH

Beetroot and horseradish are a great combination, given an extra dimension here with the butter beans and sausages. A great colour contrast as well as a great flavour contrast. You can make this perfectly successfully for one – just halve the quantities and slightly reduce the cooking time. You will have half a tin of butter beans left over but they are great in either soup or a salad. | Serves 2

---

1 tbsp olive oil

1 small onion, finely sliced

4 large fairly coarse pork sausages cut in thick rounds – you can use good British bangers or a coarse French, Spanish or Italian sausage, all of which tend to be even more flavoursome

1 medium-large raw beetroot, coarsely grated

200ml/7fl oz vegetable stock

1 x 200g tin butter beans, drained

1 tbsp fresh grated horseradish

2 tbsp soya or oat 'cream' or low fat plain yogurt

juice of approx 1/2 lemon

sea salt and freshly ground black pepper

---

Heat the oil in a wide, heavy pan. Add the onion and sausages and fry both fairly briskly for 5-10 minutes till both are gently browning.

Add the grated beetroot, stir well, then add the stock. Stir well, cover and simmer gently for 10 minutes or until the sausages are cooked – the beetroot should still have some 'crunch'.

Empty the beans with their liquid into a small pan and heat gently.

Meanwhile, mix the horseradish with the cream or yogurt and lemon juice and seasoning to taste. Drain the beans and toss them in the horseradish dressing.

Serve the beans with sausage and beetroot – a great red and white meal.

You do not really need another vegetable, but if you felt you did you could steam some broccoli or finish with some nice green leaves.

> You can buy fresh horseradish root but it is not often available and very hard to peel and grate. However, you can also buy freshly grated horseradish in jars which keeps really well in the fridge. Half a teaspoon can always be relied on to give a lift to a dressing, works really well as a dip, is great in a sandwich and can be added as a seasoning to a soup or a sauce which is struggling for flavour.

# POULTRY AND GAME

CHICKEN WITH ANCHOVY AND CAULIFLOWER

OVEN-BAKED CHICKEN WITH GINGER AND YELLOW SPLIT PEAS – AND CHICKEN SOUP

CHICKEN WITH OKRA

CHICKEN OR TURKEY BREASTS WITH ORANGE AND ARTICHOKE HEARTS

CHICKEN AND APPLE SALAD

CHICKEN SALAD WITH PUMPKIN OIL

DUCK WITH GINGER AND WATER CHESTNUTS

# CHICKEN WITH ANCHOVY AND CAULIFLOWER

This is the simplest but the tastiest of chicken dishes. I made it with cauliflower (which somehow goes particularly well with anchovies) but you could use broccoli if you prefer.

Since you are only using chicken portions you can make just a single portion. The remains of the anchovies will sit very happily in their oil in their tin in the fridge for days waiting to be used as a seasoning with beef, or in an omelette or as an alternative to salt in a salad dressing. The rest of the cauliflower can be used as a vegetable, turned into soup or used to dip into a pot of hummus or guacamole. | Serves 1 (double the quantity for 2)

---

1 large or 2 small chicken joints – breast or thigh/drumstick

2-3 anchovies from a small tin of anchovies in olive oil

½ small cauliflower

½ lemon

freshly ground black pepper

---

Skin the chicken joints and dry on kitchen paper.

Tip a tablespoon of the oil from the anchovies oil into a pan just big enough to hold the chicken, then chop the anchovies small and add them to the oil.

Fry gently for a couple of minutes to break up the anchovies.

Add the chicken and fry briskly on all sides for several minutes or until nicely browned. You may need to add a little extra olive oil depending on how much you managed to get out of the can.

When the chicken is nicely tanned all over, reduce the heat and cover the pan tightly with a lid. Cook gently for at least 15 minutes or until the chicken is cooked through.

Meanwhile, break up the cauliflower into florets and steam for around 5 minutes or until it is cooked but still slightly crunchy.

Remove the lid from the chicken and squeeze over the juice from ¼ of the lemon. Save the remaining ¼ in case you would like an extra squeeze of lemon juice when you taste the dish.

Arrange the chicken with the cauliflower on a warmed plate and pour over the juices from the pan.

Grind over some black pepper and serve at once with a green vegetable.

> Cauliflower is one of those vegetables, like beetroot, which you either love or hate, although many people hate it because they find it very indigestible. However, it is very low in carbohydrates, even though it has an almost starchy texture, so only rates 2 on the Glycaemic Load. Moreover, it contains useful amounts of protein, thiamin, riboflavin, niacin, magnesium, phosphorus, dietary fibre, vitamin C, vitamin K, vitamin B6, folate, pantothenic acid, potassium and manganese…

# CHICKEN WITH OKRA

This is a very easy, quick and colourful dish that works very well just for one – double up if there are two of you. | Serves 1

---

1 tbsp sunflower oil
1 chicken joint, breast or thigh or drumstick as you prefer
2 pieces okra, topped and tailed and chopped roughly
2 baby sweet corns, halved
1 medium courgette, sliced thickly
½ small (200g) can chopped tomatoes
4 tbsp rough red wine or vegetable stock
½ tsp dried marjoram
salt, pepper and a good squeeze of lemon juice

---

In the oil, briskly fry the chicken on all sides till they start to tan. Add the okra, corn and courgettes (zucchini) and continue to fry till the vegetables have also taken on a little colour. Add the tomatoes, the red wine or stock, marjoram and seasoning. Bring to the boil, cover and simmer gently for 20 minutes or till the chicken is quite cooked. Add lemon juice and seasoning to taste before serving.

Serve on its own or with rice and a salad if you are really hungry.

> Okra is a great vegetable for diabetics as the slightly gluey juices are very good for helping to regulate blood sugar. Even better, it is very nutritious containing significant amounts of folic acid, calcium, fibre, iron, vitamin A, vitamin C, potassium and magnesium.

# OVEN-BAKED CHICKEN WITH GINGER AND YELLOW SPLIT PEAS – AND CHICKEN SOUP

This is a great one-pot meal, good at any time of year but especially so in winter. And it provides you with a built-in second meal. | Serves 2

---

175g/6oz yellow split peas

1 tbsp olive oil

1 leek, trimmed and sliced

2 cloves garlic, peeled and sliced

15-25g/½-1oz knob of fresh ginger (depending on how much you like ginger) peeled and cut into matchsticks – or, if you cannot get fresh ginger, 1-2 heaped tsp ground ginger

½ tsp Herbes de Provence

½ small chicken, organic if possible, cut through the back so in one piece

180ml/6floz chicken stock (made from the giblets if your chicken was organic and came with giblets)

sea salt and 1 tsp black peppercorns

2 rashers back bacon

1 bouquet garni

---

Soak the peas for 3-4 hours in cold water. Strain off the water, and put the peas in a pot covered with fresh cold water. Bring to the boil and simmer for 30 minutes. Strain off the water and set the peas aside.

In a pan big enough to hold the chicken lying flat heat the oil and add the leek, garlic and ginger, if you are using fresh. Fry gently, stirring regularly, for 10 minutes or until they are quite soft.

Add the split peas, the ground ginger if you are using that, and the stock with the herbs, a little salt and the peppercorns.

Place the chicken in the pan, cut side down, so that it sinks into the peas and the stock. Cover and simmer gently for 40 minutes.

Meanwhile, heat the oven to 180C/350F/Gas mark 4.

> If you are not able to buy a half chicken, buy a whole one. With a scissors and a knife you should be able to cut it in half, even if it is a bit untidy. Use half for this dish and just freeze the other half for future use.

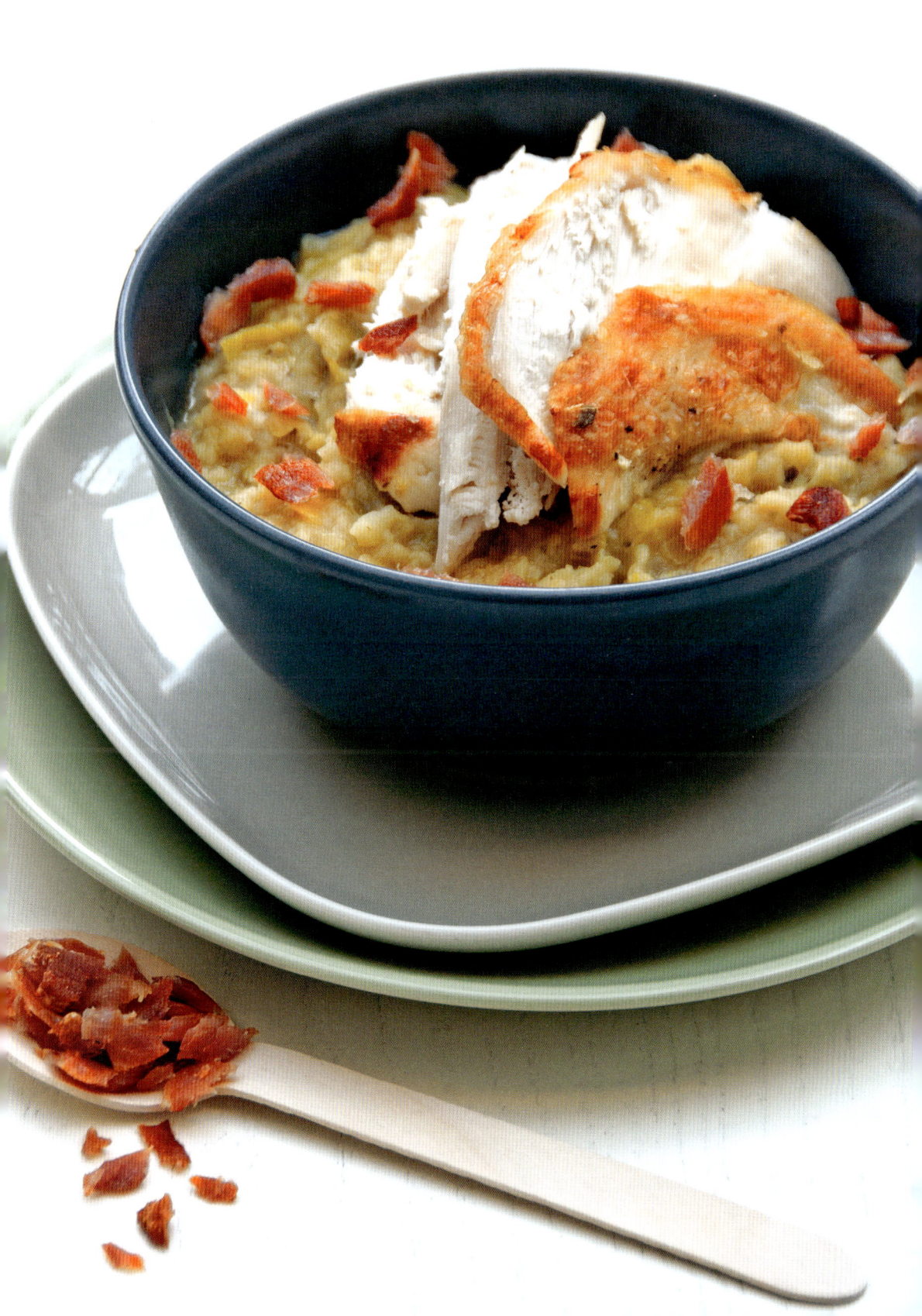

Remove the lid from the pot and cover the top of the chicken with the bacon rashers. Bake, uncovered, for a further 40 minutes to allow the top of the chicken and the bacon to get brown and crisp.

Remove the chicken from the pot to carve. Use a slotted spoon to serve the peas with the chicken and a green vegetable or salad.

When the meal is over, strip any remaining chicken from the carcass and return the flesh to the pot. Add another 300ml/½ pint of stock or water and the bouquet garni, bring back to the boil and simmer for a further 45-60 minutes to make the most delicious soup for the next day.

# CHICKEN AND APPLE SALAD

The original of this recipe came from Joan Cromwell's (wife of Oliver) own cookbook – and was decorated with the bones of the chicken… I don't think you need to go that far – but the combination is delicious. | Serves 1 (double the quantity for 2)

---

100-150g/4-6oz cooked chicken, cut into fingers

grated peel and juice of ½-1 lemon

½ small tart eating apple, cut in small dice (skin on)

1 shallot or half small onion, peeled and finely chopped

several sprigs fresh parsley or watercress, roughly chopped

sea salt and freshly ground black pepper

1 tbsp olive oil

extra watercress or leaves

---

In a bowl mix the chicken, lemon peel, apple, onion and parsley or watercress. Sprinkle to taste with sea salt and pepper then add the lemon juice to taste and olive oil and mix well.

Serve with extra watercress leaves.

# CHICKEN OR TURKEY BREASTS WITH ORANGE AND ARTICHOKE HEARTS

You can buy quite small pieces of turkey in most supermarkets now – just enough for two – if you want a change from chicken. The sauce goes equally well with both birds.

Serve with new potatoes or mashed ordinary and sweet potatoes and a green vegetable such as broccoli or spinach. | Serves 2

---

225g/8oz boneless turkey fillets or pieces or two chicken breasts

stock ingredients – a small onion, ½ carrot, 2 mushrooms, stalk of fresh parsley or dried, bouquet garni, bay leaf, some black peppercorns

1 tbsp olive oil

1 medium onion, peeled and very finely sliced

1 small stalk celery, chopped small

1 scant dessertspoon flour

4 artichoke hearts, freshly cooked, frozen or tinned – well drained and halved or quartered

2 small oranges

salt and pepper

---

Put the turkey pieces or chicken breasts with the stock ingredients and 300ml/½ pint water in a pan and bring them slowly to the boil. Simmer them gently for 20 minutes or until the meat is just cooked then remove the meat and strain and reserve the stock.

Meanwhile, heat the oil in a pan and slowly cook the onions and celery till they are soft but not coloured. Add the flour and cook for a minute or two. Then gradually add 150ml/¼ pint of the reserved stock, the rind and juice of one orange and the artichoke hearts.

Cook all together for a couple of minutes, then add the turkey pieces or chicken breasts and reheat gently.

Cut the remaining orange in segments and use to decorate the dish.

> Artichoke hearts are a great way to add interest to a dish as they have a very distinct flavour of their own and are very versatile: they can be used in a hot dish like this, a salad or a dip. They also have very small amounts of fat but high levels of fibre, vitamins B6, C and K, folate, magnesium, potassium, copper, manganese, niacin, iron and phosphorus. Fresh globe artichokes are delicious but quite seasonal but, fortunately, tinned and frozen are available all year round and are easier to use if you are incorporating them into a dish rather than eating them on their own.

# CHICKEN SALAD WITH PUMPKIN OIL

The pumpkin oil and balsamic vinegar combine to make a really delicious dressing for the chicken. If you had treated yourself to a roast chicken and had lots of chicken meat over, this would be a great way to 'use it up'.

Serve with new potatoes and a cucumber salad. | Serves 2

---

1 tbsp olive oil
1 medium onion, very finely sliced
175-225g/6-8oz cooked chicken breast and thigh meat
sea salt and freshly ground black pepper
1 tbsp balsamic vinegar
2 generous tbsp toasted pumpkin seed oil
baby spinach and pink chicory leaves
nasturtiums to decorate (optional)

---

Heat the oil in a heavy, wide pan then add the sliced onion and stir thoroughly so that the onion is well broken up. Fry VERY gently, over a very low heat, for 30 minutes. The onion should very gradually change colour and dry out but must not burn.

Slice the chicken meat and lay ½ out in a pie dish.

Grind over a little sea salt and black pepper and sprinkle over ⅓ of the onion.

In a separate bowl mix the balsamic vinegar and the pumpkin oil and spoon ½ over the chicken.

Lay another layer of chicken in the bowl and repeat the procedure. You should have ⅓ of the onion left – lay aside to decorate the dish at the end.

Leave the chicken to marinate for 3-4 hours.

To serve, arrange the spinach leaves and chicory in a dish. Spoon over the chicken, pouring any remaining marinade over the top. Sprinkle over the remaining onion and serve with new potatoes.

Balsamic vinegar has become all the rage over the last few years and, as a result, much of what is on sale is of very inferior quality and often sweetened with sugar. Real balsamic vinegar is slightly sweet but the sweetness derives from the long aging of the grape pressings in different wooden kegs – chestnut, cherry wood, ash, mulberry and juniper – and is rich and complex in flavour. It should be used very sparingly and in such a dish as this that is very low in both fat and carbohydrate, can certainly be included in the diabetic menu.

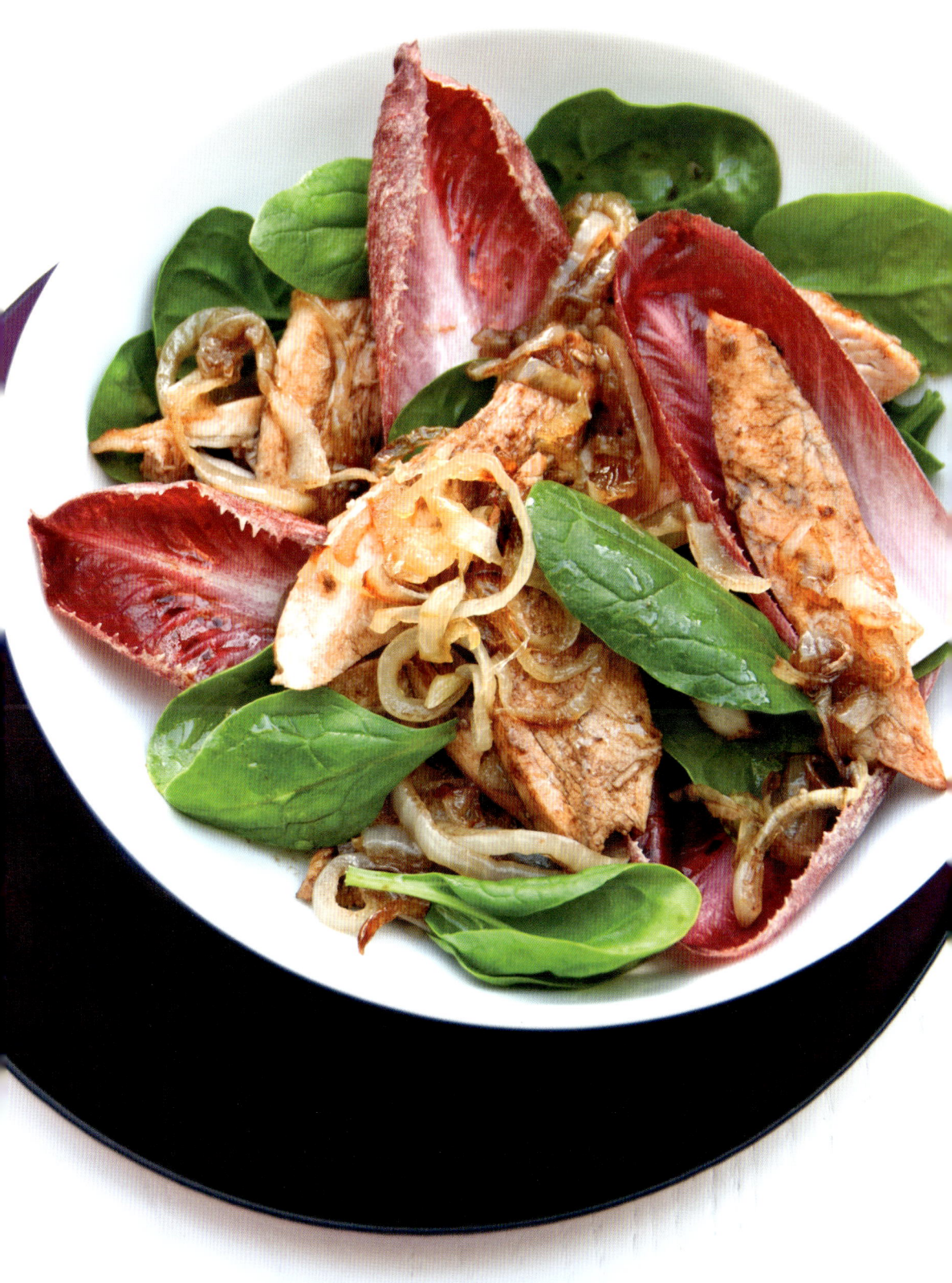

# DUCK WITH GINGER AND WATER CHESTNUTS

Ducks have less meat on them than chickens so, if you would like to have some cold duck over, you might wish to buy a whole small duck. Alternatively, you can just buy duck breasts, available in most supermarkets, and so can make the dish for one or two people. I have given the recipe for one; just double the ingredients for two.

The water chestnuts add a lovely fresh 'crunch', a nice contrast to the richness of the duck.

Serve the duck with mashed roots and a green vegetable such as broccoli, green beans or spinach. | Serves 1

---

1 duck breast with skin

1 scant tbsp olive oil

small piece of peeled root ginger, 15–25g/½–1oz, cut into thin matchsticks

125g tin water chestnuts in water

4 tbsp fresh orange juice

salt and pepper

---

Heat the oven to 190C/375F/Gas mark 5.

Prick the skin of the duck breast to release the fat. Put the breast skin side up on a rack and roast for 25 minutes.

If you do not want to heat an oven for this you can also achieve the same result if you have an electric frying pan or multicooker. If you have a small rack, place the breast on the rack and 'roast' as above.

When the duck is done, heat the oil in a small pan and add the ginger. Cook gently for a few minutes then add the water chestnuts, halved horizontally, and two tablespoons of the water from the tin.

Remove the duck from the oven and discard the fat. Add the duck to the pan along with the orange juice and simmer gently for a couple of minutes for the flavours to amalgamate. Season to taste and serve at once.

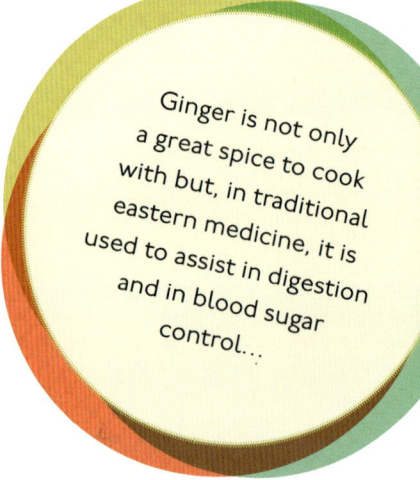

Ginger is not only a great spice to cook with but, in traditional eastern medicine, it is used to assist in digestion and in blood sugar control...

# VEGETABLES, SALADS AND VEGETARIAN DISHES

BEETROOT AND CHICKPEA OR BUTTER BEAN SALAD
CAULIFLOWER AND CASHEW NUT SALAD
CAVOLO NERO WITH BEET LEAVES
BRUSSELS SPROUT AND CELERIAC SALAD WITH HORSERADISH
RATATOUILLE WITH BUTTERNUT SQUASH
SPINACH, AVOCADO AND MOZZARELLA SALAD
CRACKED WHEAT WITH SPINACH AND PINE NUTS
PUY LENTILS WITH OKRA AND CORIANDER
CELERIAC WITH KALE AND PECAN NUTS
FENNEL AND STRAWBERRY SALAD
RED CABBAGE CASSEROLE

# BEETROOT AND CHICKPEA OR BUTTER BEAN SALAD

Both chickpeas and butter beans are low on the Glycaemic Index and both work equally well in this salad – so take your pick. The salad benefits from time to mature so if you have too much it will be fine for at least another 24 hours in the fridge. | Serves 2

---

1 raw beetroot, peeled and grated
400g tin chickpeas or butter beans, drained
3 spring onions, trimmed and chopped
1 dessertspoon soy sauce
1 dessertspoon vinegar (of your choice)
2 tbsp olive oil or 1 tbsp each olive and pumpkin oil
freshly ground black pepper

---

Mix the grated beetroot thoroughly with the chickpeas and the spring onions. Add the soy sauce, vinegar, oils and pepper and mix again thoroughly.

Cover the dish and heat for 1 minute in a microwave or tip them into a saucepan and warm gently for 2-3 minutes. Warming the chickpeas and beetroot helps them to absorb the dressing. Set aside for 2-3 hours but do not chill. Mix again thoroughly before serving.

> Tinned legumes tend to have a higher glycaemic rating than freshly cooked so if you have the time, it is better to cook your own. However, this does often mean that you have to soak them overnight first so will include some planning ahead. However, you should not stress about this as the increase for canned is only a matter of a few points still leaving both beans in the lower end of the table.

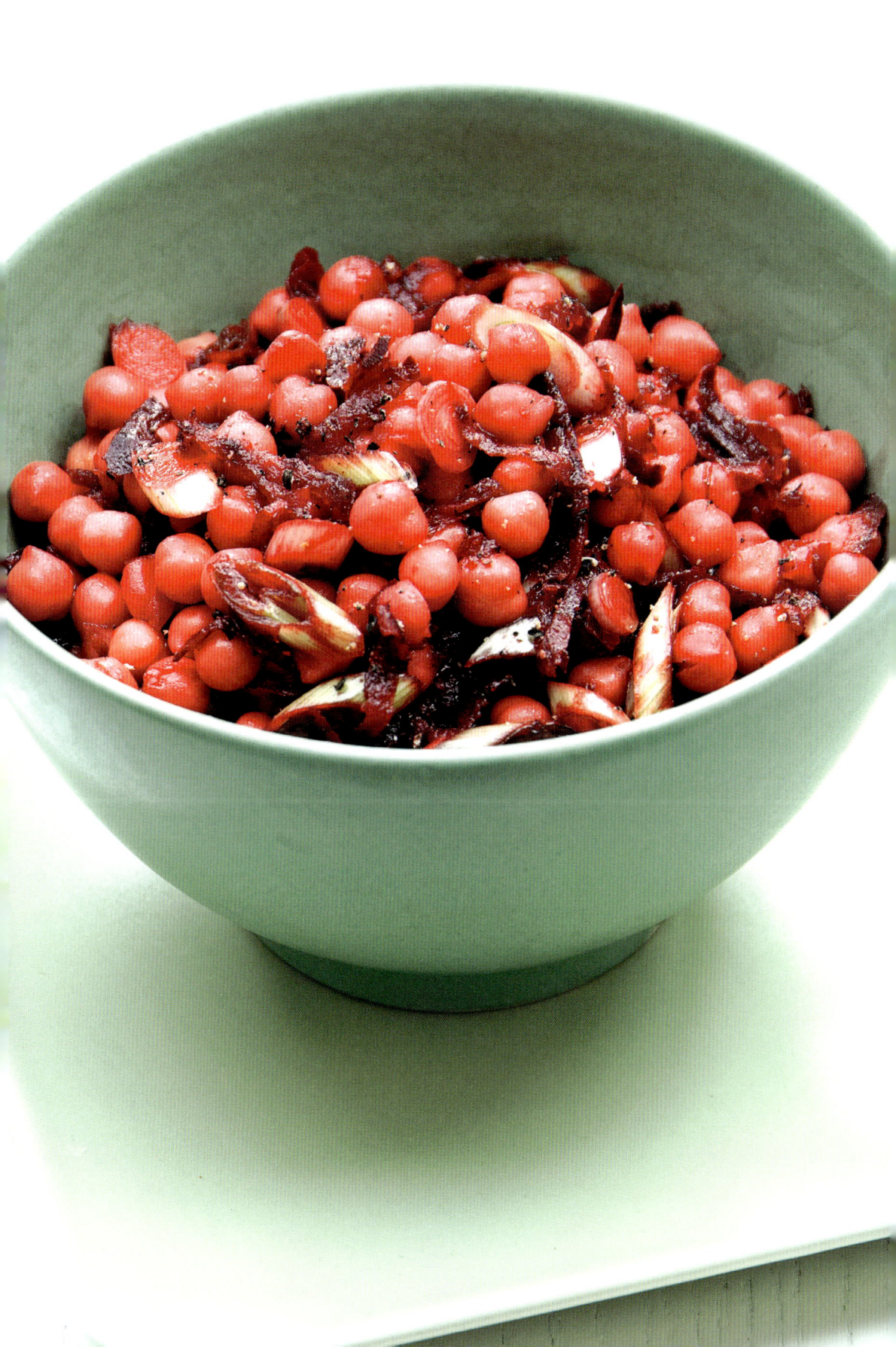

# CAULIFLOWER AND CASHEW NUT SALAD

Very simple – but delicious – and sustaining. | Serves 2

---

½ medium cauliflower broken into florets

50g/2oz roasted, salted cashews

1-2 tbsp olive oil

juice ½-1 lemon

4 sprigs parsley, chopped

---

Steam the cauliflower florets for 5-10 minutes or till they are just cooked without being mushy. Turn into a dish, mix in the nuts and sprinkle with the oil and lemon juice. Season with salt and freshly ground pepper if it needs it – if you are using salted nuts, it probably will not. Sprinkle with the parsley and serve warm or at room temperature.

*All nuts, including cashews, are very low in terms of Glycaemic Load and although they are calorific they are very nutritious – and, of course, delicious.*

# CAVOLO NERO WITH BEET LEAVES

This is a seriously nutritious salad – even more so if you can find some fresh beetroot which are still attached to their stalks and leaves as the leaves are even more laden with nutrients than the beets themselves. If you can, use the beetroots for the beetroot and chickpea salad on page 98 or the sausages with beetroot and horseradish on page 86.

If you have leftovers, they work well as a salad, especially with something relatively bland like a hard or soft boiled egg. | Serves 2

---

1 tbsp olive oil

1 small onion, peeled and sliced

½ large cooking apple, Bramley if possible, wiped and chopped small, with its skin on

sea salt

175g/6 oz Cavolo Nero

75g/3oz curly kale

75g/3oz beet greens with stalks, if you can find them – if not, double up the curly kale

2 tbsp water

sea salt and freshly ground black pepper

---

Heat the oil in a deep pan and add the onion and apple with a pinch of salt to help prevent it burning. Fry gently for 5-8 minutes or until the onion is quite soft – but watch it carefully as it will burn very easily.

Wash all the greens and remove any coarse stalks from the cavolo nero and the kale. Shake dry, leaving a fair amount of water on the leaves, then chop roughly.

Add to the onion mix, cover and cook gently for 5-10 minutes or until the greens are cooked but retain a little crunch. If they appear to be drying up, add a little water – the mixture should be moist without being wet.

Season to taste before serving.

> All these dark green leaves can taste quite bitter, no matter how nutritious they may be – which is where the apple comes in. Even a quite sharp apple such as a Bramley, takes the bitter edge off the leaves.

# BRUSSELS SPROUT AND CELERIAC SALAD WITH HORSERADISH

People rarely use Brussels sprouts raw which always seems a shame to me as they have a very delicate flavour and do not get that terrible 'school cabbage' smell which so often accompanies cooked sprouts. There is quite a lot of 'chewing' in a raw Brussels sprout so this is a filling salad. | Serves 1 (double quantities for 2)

---

50g/2oz Brussels sprouts, trimmed and finely sliced
50g/2oz celeriac root, peeled and coarsely grated
juice 1 lemon
1 level tsp grated horseradish
1 heaped tbsp mayonnaise
sea salt and freshly ground black pepper
1-2 tbsp boiling water
approx 25g/1oz either fresh rocket or lamb's lettuce

---

Mix the finely sliced Brussels with the grated celeriac and sprinkle on the lemon juice to stop the celeriac browning.

In a bowl, mix the horseradish with the mayonnaise, season with salt and pepper and thin with the boiling water. Use to dress the salad.

Once dressed, adjust the seasoning to taste and add more lemon juice if you feel it needs it.

Just before serving, mix in the rocket or lamb's lettuce.

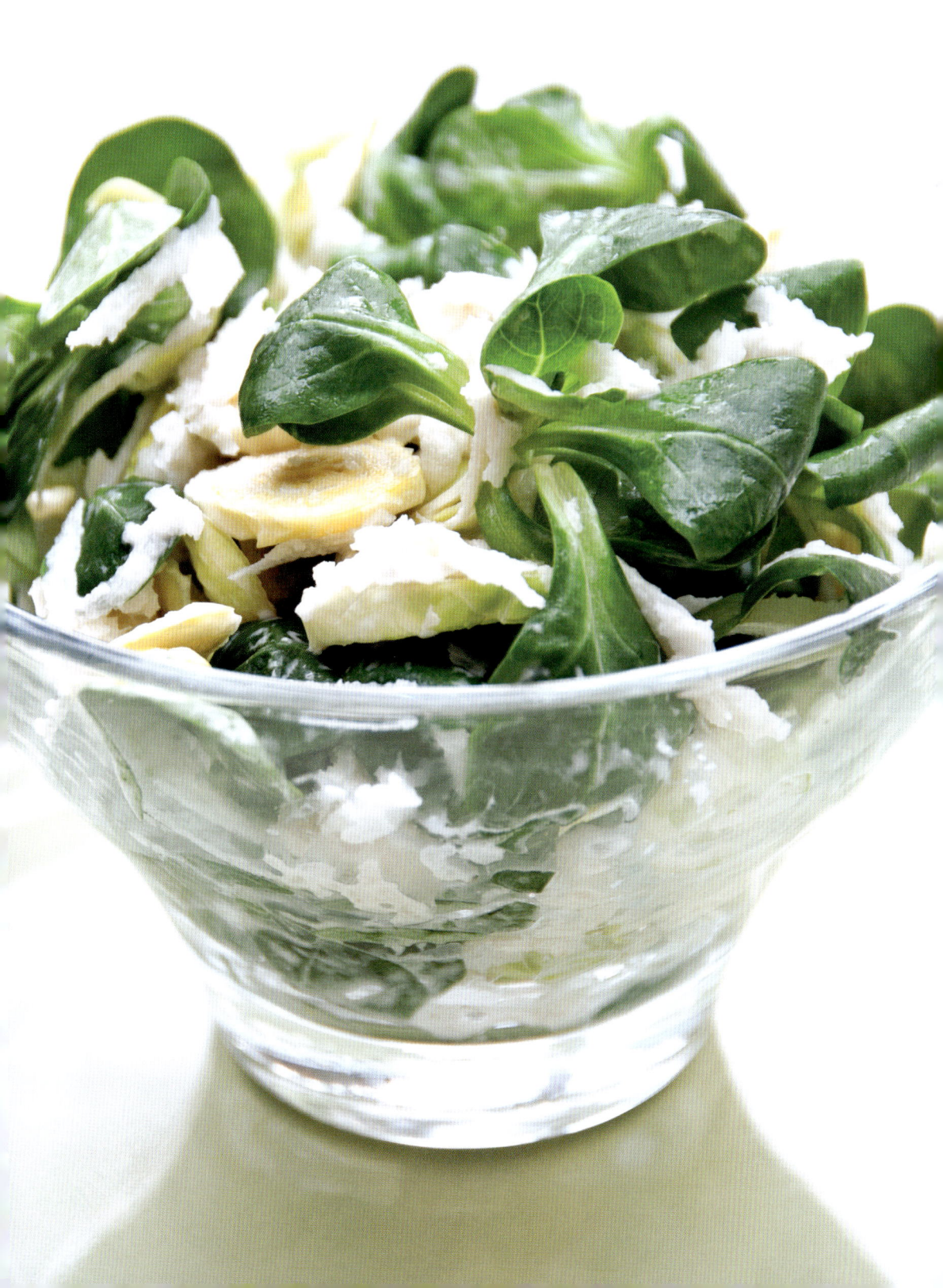

# RATATOUILLE WITH BUTTERNUT SQUASH

Adding the butternut squash to a ratatouille gives it an extra dimension in terms of both flavour and texture. You can use it as a vegetable or, for a complete vegetarian meal, cover the top with a crushed pack of crisps mixed with some grated cheese and toast lightly under the grill.

The ratatouille keeps really well if you have some left over and can be reheated or eaten cold. | Serves 2

---

1 tbsp olive oil
1 small onion, sliced
2 small peppers, one red, one yellow, sliced thinly
2 medium-large courgettes, wiped and sliced
1 small butternut squash, peeled, deseeded and diced
1 heaped tsp dried oregano or Herbes de Provence
8 cherry tomatoes, halved
sea salt and freshly ground black pepper
1 small pack of plain potato crisps (optional)
25g/1oz grated well-flavoured cheese such as Cheddar or Parmesan (optional)

---

*Squashes are not the lowest vegetables on the glycaemic tables but in this dish they are combined with vegetables which do not feature at all so the overall profile of the dish will be very acceptable.*

In a heavy pan heat the oil and add the onion and peppers. Fry fairly gently for 5-10 minutes or until they are starting to soften.

Add the courgettes, squash and herbs and continue to fry, slightly more briskly, for a further 5 minutes.

Add the tomatoes and some seasoning.

Cover the pan and reduce the heat. Cook gently for 15-20 minutes or until the squash and courgettes are cooked.

Remove the lid and, if there is too much liquid, continue to cook gently for a further 5 minutes uncovered. Season to taste.

If you wish to top it, crush the crisps and mix them with the cheese.

Transfer the ratatouille to a warmed flattish dish and sprinkle over the crisps and cheese. Brown for a couple of minutes under a hot grill but do not burn.

# SPINACH, AVOCADO AND MOZZARELLA SALAD

Such a simple salad but such a delicious one – perfect for lunch with that chilled glass of Chardonnay. | Serves 2

---

2 handfuls fresh spinach leaves – preferably mature leaves rather than the 'baby' leaves which have very little flavour

¼ bulb of fresh fennel, sliced thinly

½ young leek, sliced thinly

handful alfalfa or other favourite sprouted seeds

1 ripe avocado

1 ball buffalo mozzarella

1 level tbsp pine nuts

several sprigs of fresh basil

sea salt and freshly ground black pepper

juice 1 lemon

2-3 tbsp virgin olive oil

---

Tear up the spinach leaves in the bottom of a serving dish.

Sprinkle over the sliced fennel and leek and the seeds.

Peel the avocado and slice lengthways – arrange over the leaves.

Slice the mozzarella and lay out in the middle of the dish.

Sprinkle over the pine nuts then decorate with the basil leaves, both chopped and whole.

Grind over some sea salt and lots of black pepper, then pour over the lemon juice and the oil.

Serve at once.

*Avocados have a negligible Glycaemic Load but loads of vitamin C (among other worthwhile nutrients) and are both digestible and delicious. Combined with sprouted seeds which are not only loaded with vitamin C but with vitamin K, riboflavin, folate, magnesium, phosphorus, zinc, copper, manganese, protein, vitamin A, thiamin, pantothenic acid, calcium and iron, you should feel a new person after this meal!*

# CRACKED WHEAT WITH SPINACH AND PINE NUTS

This recipe originally came from a Roman cookery book (we are talking ancient Rome here) and is an unusual and tasty combination – although I have added to it over the years. | Serves 2

2 tbsp olive oil
50g/2oz okra, topped and tailed and cut in rounds
½ scant tsp ground cumin
50g/2oz button mushrooms, sliced
50g/2oz fresh spinach, washed and chopped
3 heaped tbsp crcked or bulgar wheat
3-7 tbsp boiling water
4 tbsp dry white wine
25g/1oz raisins
50g/2oz mangetout, chopped in half
15 g/½oz pine nuts
salt and pepper
juice ¼-½ lemon

Heat the oil in a pan and gently cook the okra and the cumin for a couple of minutes. Add the mushrooms and spinach and continue to cook for a further few minutes till both are somewhat wilted.

Meanwhile, spoon the boiling water over the cracked wheat in a bowl and leave to swell – approximately 5 minutes.

Add the cracked wheat with the wine and raisins to the pan and cook for a further few minutes.

Meanwhile, lightly steam the mangetout so that they are partially cooked but still crunchy.

Add the mangetout and pine nuts to the wheat and spinach mixture and season to taste with salt, pepper and lemon juice. Serve at once.

*While bulgar wheat is not particularly low on the Glycaemic Index, it is not high either, so it is fine combining it with very low GI foods such as the other vegetables, and especially the okra whose mucilaginous texture helps blood sugar control.*

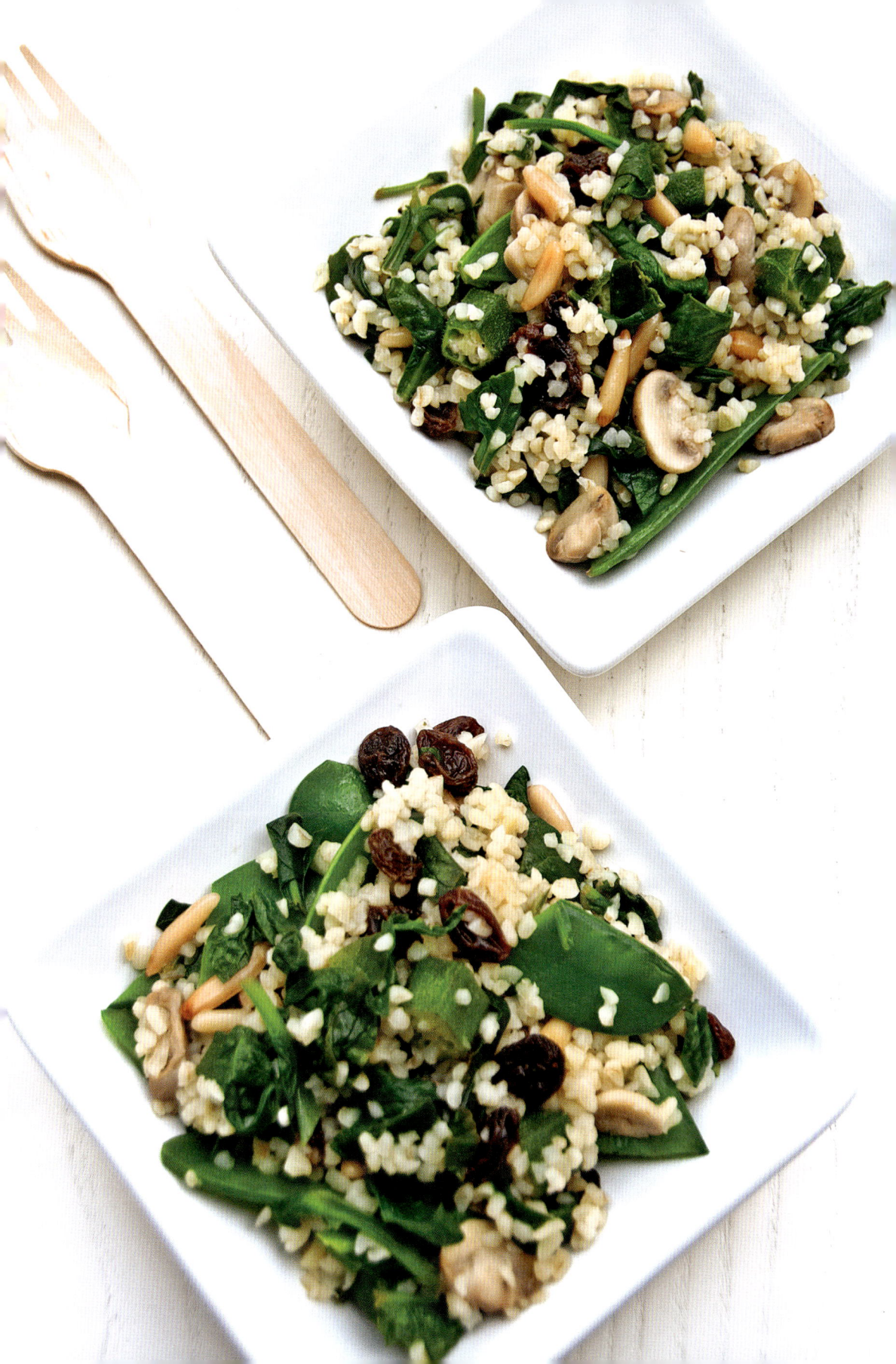

# PUY LENTILS WITH OKRA AND CORIANDER

This is a very 'lentily' looking dish (good both warm and at room temperature) but it is seriously delicious. Because it keeps very well it is worth making enough for two even if you are on your own as it will taste, if anything, even better the following day. | Serves 2

---

1 tbsp olive oil

1 small onion, peeled and chopped quite finely

1-2 large cloves garlic, peeled and finely sliced

sea salt

50g/2oz okra, topped and tailed and sliced into rounds

150g/5oz Puy lentils

3 bay leaves

400ml/14floz vegetable stock

freshly ground black pepper

juice 1 lemon

handful of fresh coriander, roughly chopped

---

Heat the oil in a heavy pan and add the onion and garlic with a pinch of salt to stop them burning. Fry gently for 5-10 minutes or until they are quite soft. Add the okra, continue to fry for a minute or two longer then add the lentils and bay leaves. Stir well to make sure they are well amalgamated then add the stock. Bring back to the boil, lower the heat and simmer, covered for 15 minutes. Then uncover and continue to simmer for a further 5-10 minutes or until the lentils are just cooked but still retain some texture and the liquid is virtually all absorbed. If they look as though they are drying out, add a little more liquid. Season to taste with salt and freshly ground black pepper.

Leave to cool to room temperature but do not chill (unless you want to store them).

To serve, add the lemon juice to taste and the fresh coriander – mix well and season further if needed.

> Lentils are generally seen to be an excellent food for diabetics and some people choose to start the day, Indian fashion, with a dish of lentils – an eastern version of porridge. This particular dish of course also includes okra, another excellent diabetic food.

# CELERIAC WITH KALE AND PECAN NUTS

This dish can be served as a vegetable with a roast or as a vegetarian dish on its own. The contrast between the pale celeriac and the dark kale works well both in terms of looks and flavour. | Serves 1 (double quantities for 2)

250g/9oz celeriac root – about ½ a small celeriac
pinch ground nutmeg
sea salt and freshly ground black pepper
small knob of butter or 1 tbsp goat, soya or oat cream
75g/3oz curly kale
1 tbsp olive oil
25g/1oz pecan nuts, lightly toasted under the grill

Heat the oven to 180C/350F/Gas mark 4.

Trim the celeriac, cut in cubes and steam until soft. Remove from the steamer and purée in a food processor with the butter or cream. Season to taste with the salt, pepper and nutmeg. Meanwhile, trim the kale of all stalks, chop it small and steam till just cooked. Mix the kale into the celeriac, turn onto a warmed serving plate and sprinkle the toasted pecan nuts over the top.

> Pecans are another really delicious food which is 'free' on the Glycaemic Index – and filled with nutrition. Often used as an alternative to walnut they actually have a rather sweeter, smoother flavour which is really accentuated by roasting or toasting.

# FENNEL AND STRAWBERRY SALAD

The arrival of real home strawberries is always worth celebrating so here is a slightly unusual, but delicious salad for early May. | Serves 1 (double quantities for 2)

---

½ bulb fennel

1 scant tbsp plain yogurt – cow, sheep, goat or soya

juice ¼–½ lemon

2-3 mint leaves, fresh if possible

4-5 strawberries, halved or quartered depending on their size

---

Trim the fennel and slice it thinly. Blanch it in boiling water for 3 minutes, cool under cold water and drain. Meanwhile, mix the yogurt with the lemon juice and mint leaves – add the mint leaves gradually as their flavour is very strong and can swamp the rest. You may want to add a little salt although I did not find it necessary.

Toss the fennel and the halved or quartered strawberries in the dressing and arrange on a serving dish. Decorate with some fronds of fennel.

*If you are concerned about pesticide residues in your vegetables, strawberries are the one fruit that you should always buy organic as conventionally grown strawberries are sprayed, not just once, but throughout their growing season.*

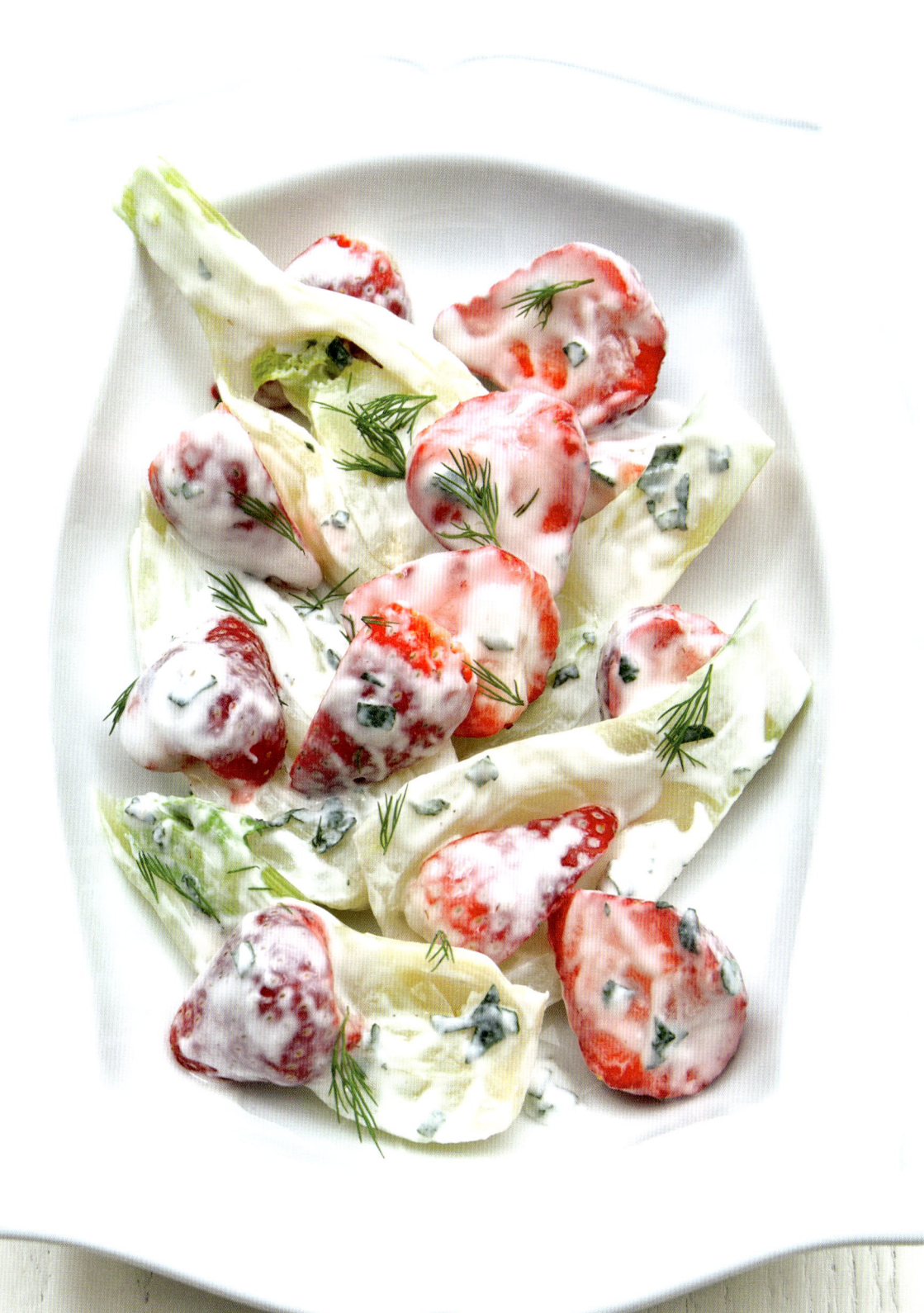

# RED CABBAGE CASSEROLE

A great winter casserole that can be used both as a vegetable and a dish on its own. It is easy to make, filling, flavoursome, low GI and nutritious… It also reheats well so it is worth making enough for two meals even if you are on your own. | Serves 2

---

1 tbsp sunflower or olive oil
1 large onion, peeled and sliced
1/3 medium red cabbage, sliced fairly thinly
2 small sweet potatoes, peeled and diced
1 small Bramley cooking apple, peeled, cored and diced
1 heaped tsp dried dill
pinch nutmeg, freshly grated if possible
1/2 tsp coriander seeds
6 tbsp water or vegetable stock
1 tbsp pumpkin seeds
1 tbsp sunflower seeds
juice 1/2 large lemon
sea salt and freshly ground black pepper

---

Heat the oil in a heavy casserole and add all the ingredients except the pumpkin seeds, sunflower seeds and lemon juice. Bring gradually to the simmer, cover and cook gently for 30 minutes or until the sweet potato is cooked through and the red cabbage is cooked but still retains some crunch. Add the pumpkin seeds, sunflower seeds and the lemon juice.

Season to taste and serve.

> Yoghurt goes really well with red cabbage and you might like to finish off the dish with a spoonful of plain live yoghurt on the top of each portion before you serve it.

# FESTIVE MEALS

# PIGEON BREASTS BRAISED WITH CHESTNUTS – OR PRUNES

Since this is a party dish I have been quite generous with the portions allowing you two pigeon breasts each. However, it is also a 'slow cook' dish and will taste better if you can cook it the day before you want to eat it to allow it to rest and the flavours to mature. I am super keen on chestnuts and would be happy to add them to every dish, but if you are not so keen, an excellent alternative with the pigeons are prunes which, although they are a dried fruit, have a surprisingly low Glycaemic Load. | Serves 2 – generously

---

1 small onion, peeled and halved
2 cloves garlic, peeled
1 small carrot, sliced thickly
1 small parsnip, scrubbed and sliced thickly
3 medium mushrooms, halved
100g/4oz piece belly pork, cut in half
2 pigeons
2 bay leaves
1-2 sprigs fresh thyme
1 large sprig parsley
½ tsp black peppercorns
150ml/¼ pint red wine plus water to cover
½ medium celeriac, peeled and diced
150g/5oz cooked chestnuts or 50g/2oz soft, stoned prunes
½ tbsp plain flour
pinch dark muscovado sugar or xylitol
sea salt

---

Put the onion, garlic, carrot, parsnip, mushrooms, belly pork, and pigeons in a heavy casserole. Lay the herbs on the top, sprinkle over the peppercorns and pour over the wine. Add enough water to just cover the pigeons.

Bring slowly to the boil, cover and simmer very gently for 2-3 hours or until the pigeon breasts are relatively soft when you spear them with a knife.

Steam the celeriac.

Remove from the heat and remove the pigeons from the pot. With a sharp knife, cut off the breasts. Set that aside and then set aside the pigeon carcases and belly pork to make soup stock later.

Strain the vegetables etc from the cooking liquids. Set the liquid aside in a cool place and once they are chilled, remove any excess fat which rises to the top.

Meanwhile, remove the herbs from the vegetable mixture and discard. Purée the vegetables with the steamed celeriac in a food processor and season to taste. Set aside.

To finish the dish, mix the flour with 50ml of the de-fatted cooking liquid to make a smooth paste. Gradually add a further 300ml/½ pint of stock, heating and stirring it as you do so until it thickens slightly. Season to taste and add a pinch of dark muscovado sugar or Xylitol if you think it needs it.

Meanwhile, halve the chestnuts.

Add the chestnuts and the reserved pigeon meat to the sauce and heat slowly.

Meanwhile, reheat the vegetable purée in a microwave or the oven and cook a green vegetable of your choice.

Serves the pigeon in its sauce with the vegetables.

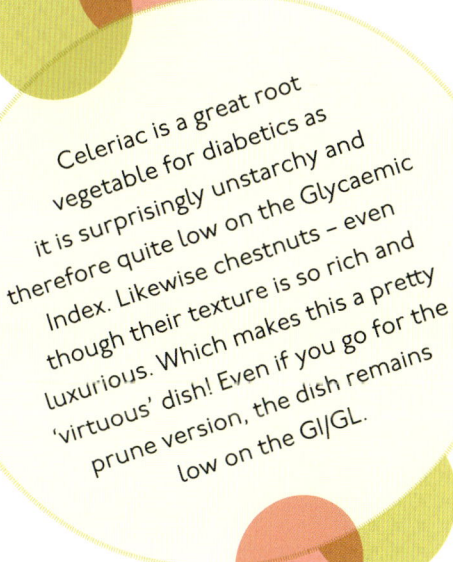

Celeriac is a great root vegetable for diabetics as it is surprisingly unstarchy and therefore quite low on the Glycaemic Index. Likewise chestnuts – even though their texture is so rich and luxurious. Which makes this a pretty 'virtuous' dish! Even if you go for the prune version, the dish remains low on the GI/GL.

# FAISANT AUX CHATAIGNES

Chestnuts seem to go particularly well with game and add a luxurious texture and taste to any dish. As with all game dishes, this is best if cooked in advance and given time to rest.
| Serves 2

---

150g/5oz fresh or tinned chestnuts
1 medium parsnip
2 tbsp olive oil
8 shallots, peeled
16 small button mushrooms, wiped
1 medium pheasant
3 bay leaves
100ml/4floz chicken or vegetable stock
100ml/4floz light red wine
sea salt and freshly ground black pepper

---

If you are using fresh chestnuts, heat the oven to 180C/350F/Gas mark 4, spread the chestnuts out on a rack and bake for 30 minutes or until they peel easily. Remove from the oven, cool slightly and peel. If you are using tinned chestnuts, drain and set aside. Scrub the parsnip and slice into thin discs. Heat 1 tbsp of the oil in a wide pan and fry the parsnip briskly for several minutes till lightly browned on both sides. Add the shallots and continue to cook for another few minutes, then remove both with a slotted spoon into a heavy casserole. Add the remaining tablespoon of oil to the wide pan and briskly fry the mushrooms for a few minutes then add to the casserole.

Stuff a couple of bay leaves inside the pheasant then place the bird on top of the vegetables. Arrange the remaining bay leaves around it then pour over the stock and the red wine. Grind over a little sea salt and black pepper. Bring slowly to the boil, then cover the casserole and reduce the heat until the pot is only just simmering. Simmer gently for one hour. Add the chestnuts and continue to cook for a further hour. Ideally, leave to 'mature' for several hours or overnight then reheat to serve with a green vegetable or salad.

NB If you cannot eat nuts, leave out the chestnuts and increase the shallots to 20 and the mushrooms to 40. Add 100g/3½oz stoned prunes when you would have added the chestnuts.

# CRAB, GINGER AND ALMOND SOUFFLÉ

I have given quantities for a fairly generous soufflé so that you can make this your main course. It will be quite rich so just serve it with some steamed fine green beans or a green salad.

Everyone gets very nervous about soufflés but they are really not hard to make as long as you put in plenty of eggs, do not cook them too fast – and eat them as soon as they come out of the oven.

You can actually make a soufflé perfectly successfully for one if you want to treat yourself. Just halve the quantities and cook for 15–20 minutes instead of 30. | Serves 2

---

25g/1oz butter
2 spring onions, finely chopped
10g/½ oz fresh ginger root, peeled and finely chopped
1 scant tbsp plain flour
2 tbsp white wine
150ml/¼ pint milk
juice ½ lemon
100g/4oz crabmeat, mixed brown and white
10g/½ oz ground almonds
salt and pepper
4 egg yolks and 5 egg whites

---

Heat the oven to 180C/350F/Gas mark 4.

Melt the butter in a pan and very gently fry the onions and ginger root till soft but not coloured. Add the flour, stir and cook for a couple of minutes, then gradually add the wine, milk and lemon juice and cook till the sauce thickens. Add the crabmeat and ground almonds, mix well and season to taste with salt and pepper. Remove from the heat, cool slightly.

Stir the egg yolks into the crab mixture.

Whisk the egg whites till they form soft peaks. Stir one third of the whites into the soufflé mixture then lightly fold in the rest. Scrape the mixture into a soufflé dish - it should ¾ fill it – and put it straight into the oven.

Cook for 30 minutes or until it is well risen and lightly browned on top.

Meanwhile, cook your vegetables or make your salad so that you are ready to serve the soufflé the minute it is cooked.

*This is a splendidly low GI dish so you can splash out on one of those yummy desserts in the next chapter.*

# NEW ORLEANS JAMBALAYA

A jambalaya is a rather exotic Caribbean stew and although it is traditionally served with rice (not good for diabetics) that is, as with so many traditional dishes, just to bulk it out and make the meat or fish go further. In fact, it works really well as a 'stew' with a 'cooling' salad.
| Serves 2

---

1 tbsp sunflower oil
2 large pork sausages, skinned
75g/3oz chorizo or spicy sausage, cubed
1 dried chilli, deseeded and cut very small
50g/2oz piece ham, cubed
1 medium onion, chopped finely
1 stick celery, chopped small
1 red pepper, chopped small
½ tbsp dried thyme
2 bay leaves
400g tin chopped tomatoes
4 tbsp chicken stock
4 large fresh or frozen prawns, peeled
4 spring onions, chopped

---

Heat the oil in a large pan and sauté the sausage meat, chorizo, chilli and the ham for a couple of minutes, then add the celery, onion and red pepper and sauté for 5 minutes.

Add the thyme and bay leaf and the tinned tomatoes. Mix well and cook for a few minutes.

Add the chicken stock, bring to the boil then simmer slowly for 10-15 minutes to allow the flavours to amalgamate.

Add the prawns, continue to cook for a couple of minutes to cook the prawns then season to taste and sprinkle over the spring onions.

Serve at once with a green salad.

*The combining of meat and fish in one dish is a particularly American habit. The Jambalaya is relatively low key – if you want to do the job properly, go for 'Surf and Turf' – steak and lobster!*

# VENISON BRAISED WITH PORT AND REDCURRANTS

This is a real winter celebration dish. Venison is a very low fat meat but that means that it can be very dry, which is why it is particularly well suited to a marinade and pot roasting. It improves with keeping so if you want to make it for one, it will be even better on the second night.

I would serve it with a celeriac purée (steamed and puréed in a food processor) and a green vegetable or salad. | Serves 2

---

2 rashers bacon, chopped fairly small
100g/4oz onions, finely chopped
50g/2oz open mushrooms, chopped finely
½ tsp dried thyme
450g/16oz piece venison, well trimmed
150ml/¼ pint port
150ml/¼ pint red wine
10g/½ oz butter
10g/½ oz flour
150ml/¼ pint water
100g/4oz redcurrants
salt and pepper

---

Put the bacon, onions, mushrooms, thyme and venison in a bowl and cover with the port and wine. Leave to marinate for up to 24 hours.

Remove the venison from the marinade and dry it on some kitchen paper. Heat the butter in a pan till sizzling and briskly fry the venison till tanned all over. Reduce the heat and add the flour, stir around for a couple of minutes then add the marinade.

Bring slowly to the boil, cover, reduce the heat and simmer very gently 1½-2 hours or until the meat is really tender.

Add the redcurrants, cook for a further five minutes then season to taste and serve with a celeriac purée and a green vegetable or salad.

> The redcurrants add a very welcome sharpness to this dish but are very low on the Glycaemic Index. Red wine has a Glycaemic Index of zero but of course port, being a sweetened wine does have a higher residual amount of sugar. However, within the context of this dish the amount will be negligible.

FESTIVE MEALS

# SALMON IN PARMA HAM

A really unusual combination – but it works very well. Serve with a green vegetable and/or a salad. I have given ingredients for two but if you want to make it for one, just halve the quantities. | Serves 2

---

1 tbsp olive oil

100g/4oz mushrooms, wiped and chopped

1 large clove garlic, peeled and sliced

2 large handfuls fresh spinach, chopped

sea salt and freshly ground black pepper

2 fillets fresh salmon

4 slices Parma ham

a little extra oil

---

Heat the oven to 180C/350F/Gas mark 4.

Heat the oil in a flattish pan and briskly fry the mushrooms and garlic for a few minutes without burning until they are just softening, then add the spinach and continue to cook for another minute or so until the spinach wilts.

Whizz this mixture in a food processor into a rough purée but do not make too smooth.

Meanwhile, skin the salmon fillets and season lightly, then grill for a few minutes on each side – they should be about two thirds cooked.

Lay the slices of Parma ham out on the counter. Spread half the mushroom mixture over the ham then place a salmon fillet at one end of the ham. Fold the other side over the top so that the fillet is enclosed.

Move this onto a piece of foil laid on a rack in a baking tray, then repeat the process with the other fillet.

Bake for 15 minutes to finish cooking the salmon and to crisp up the top layer of Parma ham.

Meanwhile cook your vegetables or make your salads.

Remove the salmon from the oven, drizzle with a little extra oil and grate over a little extra pepper. Serve at once with the vegetables or salad.

# DESSERTS

APPLE AND BERRY CRUMBLE
HOT PLUM DESSERT
COCONUT MILK CRÈME
APPLE AND CRANBERRY CLAFOUTIS
CHRISTMAS UPSIDE DOWN CAKE
HOT FRUIT SALAD
OATY STRAWBERRY OR RASPBERRY CRUMBLE
BAKED LEMON AND ALMOND CHEESECAKE
PEARS WITH CHOCOLATE AND GINGER WINE SAUCE
CHOCOLATE POTS
CHOCOLATE STRAWBERRIES

# APPLE AND BERRY CRUMBLE

This is a totally flexible recipe which uses whatever fruits you favour or are in season. You should cook the fruits before you sweeten them as different fruits will need different amounts of sweetening and with some combinations you may not need any extra sweetness at all.

If you want to avoid using any sweetener you could substitute dates as they will still provide you with sweetness but in a much more diabetic-friendly manner as it comes buried in fibre.

I suggest making enough for two as the dessert keeps well and is delicious cold. | Serves 2

---

1 Bramley cooking apple, 2 tart eating apples or other hard fruit

200g/7oz mixed berries or currants – or a combination of the two depending on what is available

4-6 tbsp water

½-1 tbsp raw cane molasses, dark molasses sugar or agave syrup or 2 fresh dates

50g/2oz rolled oats

1 level tsp each flaked almonds, pine nuts and pistachio nuts

---

Heat the oven to 180C/350F/Gas mark 4.

Wash and core the apples or other fruit. Chop them into small pieces, leaving the skin on. Trim or de-stem the currants if you are using them.

Put the fruit into a pan with the water and the dates, if you are using them. Cover and bring to the boil. Simmer for 5 minutes or until the apple is nearly cooked.

Sweeten to taste if you need to then transfer to a small pie dish.

Mix the oats with the nuts. Spread this mixture over the fruit and bake in a moderate oven for 30 minutes or until the topping is lightly browned.

Serve hot, warm or at room temperature, alone or with yogurt or cream.

> Old fashioned recipes for crumble toppings always included both fats and sugar but I think both are completely unnecessary. A good combination of cereals, nuts and seeds gives a great texture, a great flavour, a great nutritional profile and cuts out the need for any excess sugar.

# HOT PLUM DESSERT

Mixing just a few dried plums (prunes) with the fresh fruit gives you a little sugar boost without pushing up the sugar content of the dish too far. Using chickpea or gram flour gives you an unusual, slightly nuttier texture and taste than even wholewheat flour – with a lower Glycaemic Load.

Since this is another dessert which tastes good cold I am giving the recipe for two.

| Serves 2

---

225g/8oz fresh plums
25g/1oz softened/ready to eat prunes
50g/2oz butter
25g/1oz dark muscovado sugar or agave syrup
50g/2oz chickpea (gram) flour
½ level tsp baking powder
1 egg

---

Put half the plums with the prunes in a small pan. Cover and cook over a very low heat for 30 minutes, stirring regularly, until they have cooked down into a 'marmalade'.

Heat the oven to 180C/350F/Gas mark 4.

Remove the stones from the fruit mixture and spread it out in the bottom of a small oven-proof pie dish. Halve the remaining plums and remove their stones. Lay them out, cut side up, over the mixture.

Beat the butter with the sugar in an electric mixer till they are soft and fluffy. Sift the flour with the baking powder.

Beat the egg into the butter and sugar with a little flour then fold in the remaining flour.

Spoon the mixture over the plums and bake for 30-35 minutes or till a skewer comes out clean.

Either serve the pudding from the pie dish or loosen the edges and turn it out onto a serving dish. Serve warm with cream or yoghurt.

> Plums are relatively high in pectin and pectin is generally regarded as helpful for diabetics because, being a soluble fibre, it helps regulate blood sugar control. Raw apples are the richest source of pectin but plums contain useful amounts.

# COCONUT MILK CRÈME

This is one of my favourite recipes as it tastes delicious and yet is good for those trying to avoid dairy products and sugar. I have replaced the classic burnt sugar topping with toasted almonds – even better! You can make yourself a single portion whenever you feel like a treat.
| Serves 1 (double quantities for 2)

---

6 tbsp coconut milk

1 small vanilla pod or 1/4 tsp vanilla essence

1/2 tsp agave syrup (optional)

1 large egg yolk

1 level tsp nibbed almonds

---

Heat the milk with the vanilla pod or essence until just below boiling point. Remove the vanilla pod and taste. If you would like it slightly sweeter, add ½ teaspoon of agave syrup.

Whisk the egg yolk thoroughly with a fork (a whisk makes it too frothy) and, whisking all the time, add the milk. Pour into a small ramekin dish and place in a low oven, 150C/300F/Gas mark 2, for 20-30 minutes or until it is just set.

Meanwhile, lightly toast the almonds in the oven or in a dry frying pan.

When the cream has cooled slightly, spread them over the top.

Serve chilled or at room temperature, as you prefer.

> Coconut milk is naturally sweet yet has a low Glycaemic Load and although high in saturated fat this is in the form of medium chain triglycerides which are now recognised to be very helpful with weight control, atherosclerosis and cardiovascular disease and to have a slight blood-glucose lowering effect.

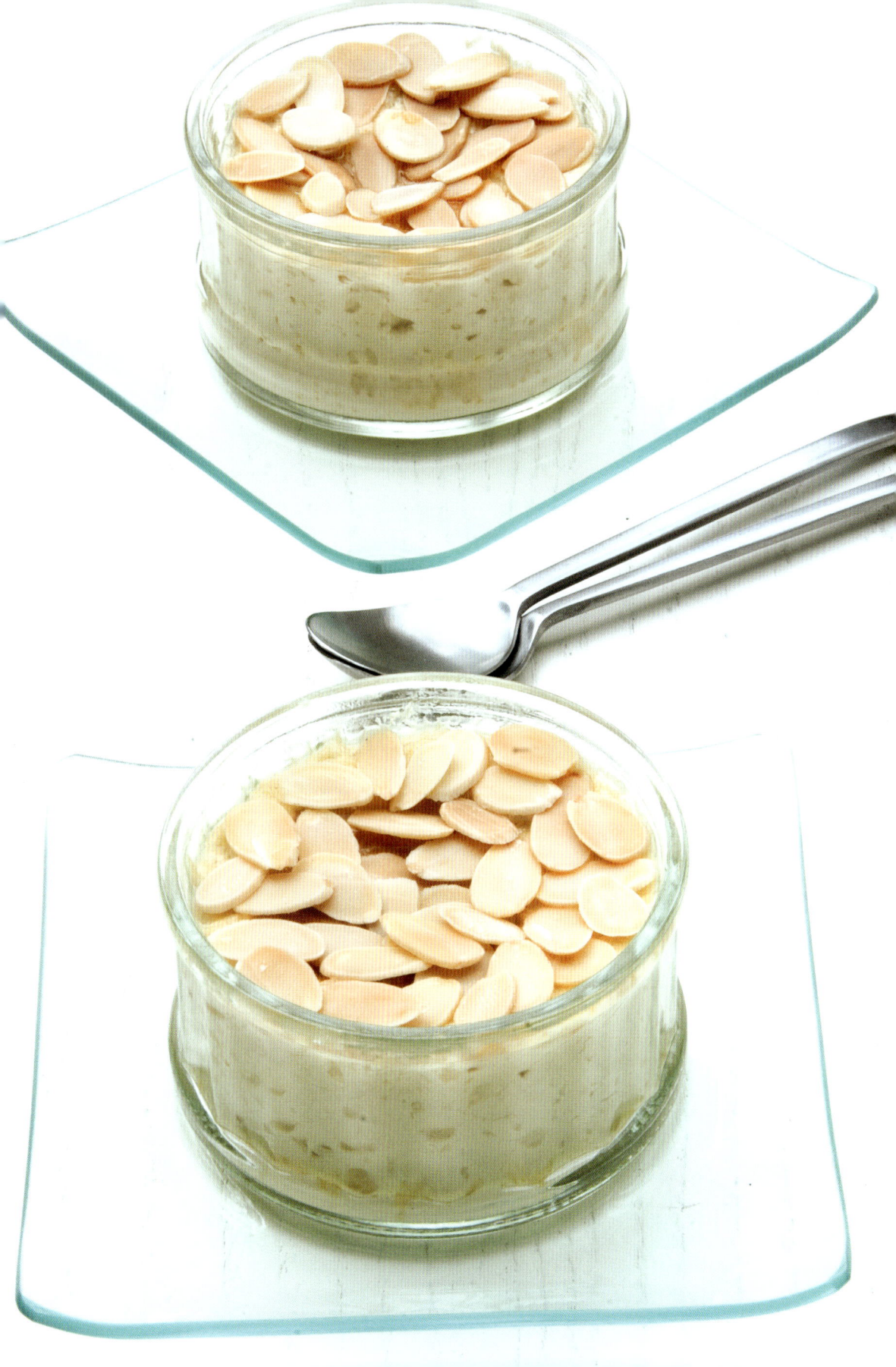

# APPLE AND CRANBERRY CLAFOUTIS

The dates, along with the little dash of liqueur, should provide enough sweetness for this dish but if you do not want to use the liqueur add ½ tsp of agave syrup to the milk. If you can get, and like, nut milk (almond or hazelnut) it gives the dish an interesting extra layer of flavour. The clafoutis tastes good cold as well as hot so I suggest you make enough for two even if you are on your own. | Serves 2

---

1 Bramley cooking apple, peeled and sliced – or 2 tart eating apples, peeled and sliced

50g/2oz fresh cranberries

2 soft dates

2 small eggs

1 tsp orange liqueur such as Grand Marnier or agave syrup

150ml/¼ pint milk – cow, unsweetened soya, oat or nut

---

Heat the oven to 180C/350F/Gas mark 4.

Turn the sliced apple into a flan dish along with the cranberries.

Stone the dates and cut them in thin slithers. Mix them into the other fruit.

Beat the eggs in a bowl and add the liqueur or agave and whichever milk you are using.

Pour over the fruit in the dish and bake, uncovered for 30-40 minutes or until the custard is set.

Serve warm or at room temperature.

> You may have noticed that cranberries can taste quite bitter. However, if you stop cooking them as soon as they start to pop you should be able to avoid this. Baking them, as in the dish above, certainly avoids it.

# CHRISTMAS UPSIDE DOWN CAKE

For those who want a hint of the Christmas spirit but cannot tolerate the sugar levels delivered by all those dried fruits in a normal Christmas pudding. The combination of flours gives it an excellent and interesting texture. It is delicious warm out of the oven – but also excellent cold as a cake. And of course you do not only have to eat it at Christmas! | Serves 2

---

1 small ripe eating apple, cored, peeled and sliced
½ tsp raisins
1 soft date, stoned and chopped
generous pinch each of ground ginger and cinnamon
mean pinch each of cloves and ground nutmeg
rind and juice ½ lemon
1 tsp brandy
50g/2oz butter or coconut oil
25g/1oz pale muscovado sugar
25g/1oz each rice flour and coarse polenta
pinch each ground ginger and cinnamon
⅓ level tsp baking powder
1 egg

---

Put the apple in a small bowl with the raisins, date, spices, lemon rind, half the lemon juice and the brandy. Stir well around until the fruit is well coated in the spices and the liquid then cover and leave to steep for 1-3 hours.

Heat the oven to 180C/350F/Gas mark 4.

Line a small loose-bottomed cake tin with foil and oil lightly. Spread the fruit mixture out over the bottom of the cake tin, flattening it out as much as possible.

Beat the butter or coconut oil with the sugar with an electric or hand whisk until light and creamy.

Sieve the rice flour with the baking powder and mix into the polenta.

With a wooden spoon, beat the egg into the butter and sugar mixture with a little flour then fold in the rest of the flour with the remaining lemon juice.

Spoon carefully into the tin and flatten out by banging the cake tin gently on the counter. Bake for 20-25 minutes or until a skewer comes out clean.

Carefully turn out onto a serving dish and then, also carefully, peel off the foil.

# HOT FRUIT SALAD

This is really an old fashioned compote and you can leave it in the fridge for weeks and just dip in when you feel inclined – the flavours get better as they mature. In some recipes you do not even cook the fruit, just leaving all to macerate in their juices.

I am giving relatively large quantities to allow you to keep it long enough to prove me right about maturing flavours. | Serves 4

---

500g/1lb mixed dried fruits of your choice (apricots, apples, prunes, large raisins, sultanas, figs, pears etc)

450ml/15floz water

4 tbsp red wine

rind of a small lemon, thinly pared

stick of cinnamon or 1 level tsp ground cinnamon

---

If the fruit is very dry, soak it overnight then drain it and discard the water. Put it in fresh water with the wine, lemon rind and cinnamon in a pan and heat gently. Simmer gently for 10-15 minutes or till it is cooked. Remove the fruit into a bowl and continue to simmer the juice gently for a further 20 minutes till it is thickened and slightly reduced. Pour it over the fruit. Serve the compote warm or cold with cream or yogurt, or with your favourite breakfast cereal.

Even though they contain a good deal of natural sugar, dried fruits have a relatively low Glycaemic Load because they also contain significant amounts of fibre and nutrients. So, provided you do not add any extra sugar, they are perfectly acceptable within a diabetic diet.

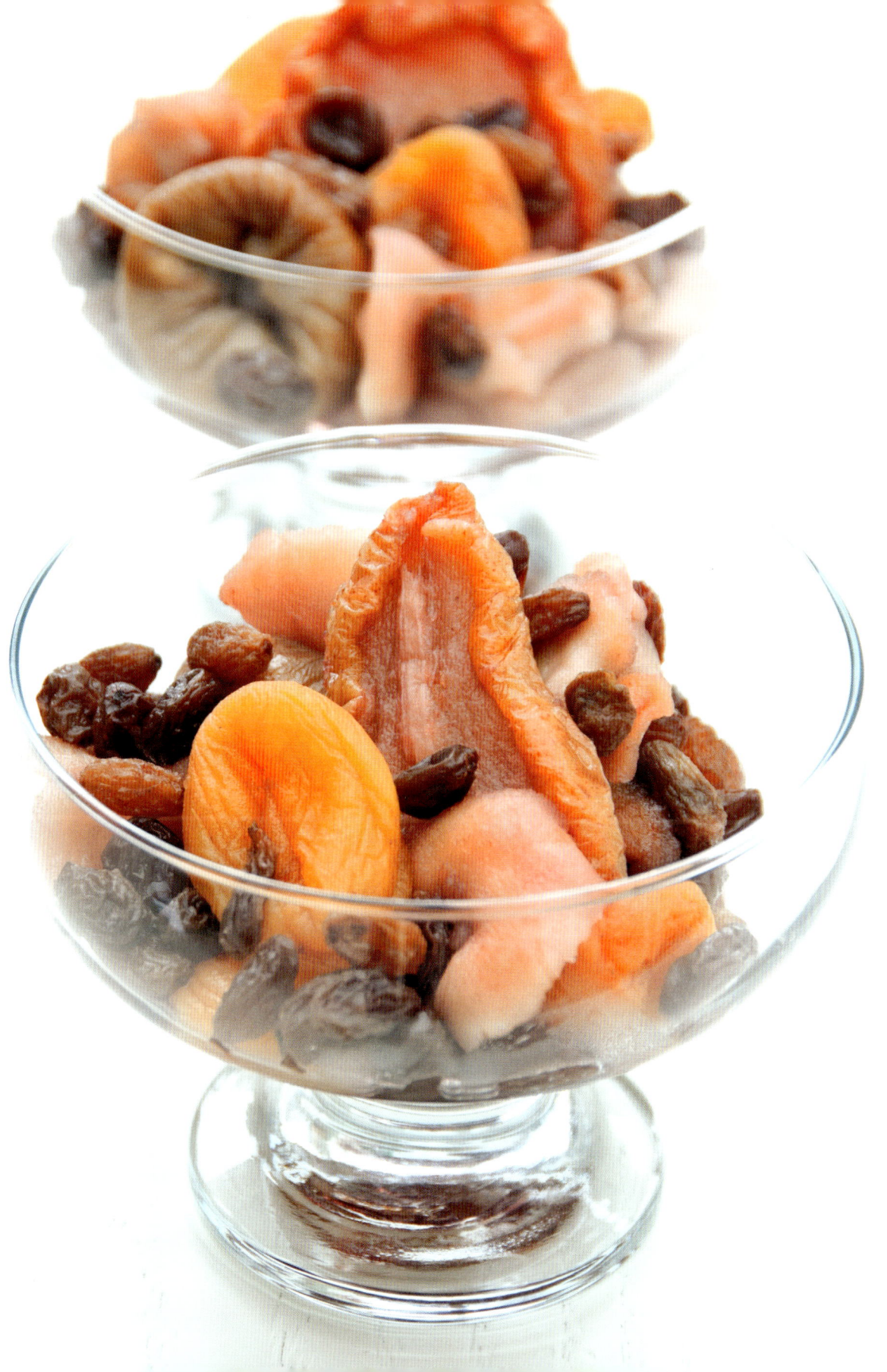

# OATY STRAWBERRY OR RASPBERRY CRUMBLE

This is a different take on a crumble – and is a great way to use up any fruit which may be a bit squashed or over ripe. It is good both hot and cold so make enough for two even if you are on your own. | Serves 2

---

25g/1oz coconut oil or butter

75g/3oz porridge oats

25g/1oz coarse polenta or wholemeal flour

1 tbsp agave syrup

250g/9oz strawberries or raspberries

1 heaped tsp arrowroot

---

Heat the oven to 180C/350F/Gas mark 4.

Melt the coconut oil or butter and mix in the oats, polenta and agave syrup. Purée half of the fruit and, if you are using strawberries, chop the rest fairly roughly.

Put the arrowroot in a small pan and add a little of the purée, stir till smooth, then add the rest of the purée. Heat gently till the sauce thickens then amalgamate it with the chopped strawberries.

Spread half of the crumble mixture over the bottom of a small shallow baking dish or flan dish – you need it to be at least 1 cm/½ inch thick. Spread the strawberry mixture over the crumble and the rest of the crumble over the strawberries.

Bake the crumble for 30 minutes. Serve warm or cold – alone or with yogurt or cream.

*Coconut oil is a good substitute for butter for the diabetic as although it is just as high in saturated fat as butter, the saturated fat in coconut oil is largely medium chain triglycerides which are helpful for weight loss and atherosclerosis as well as blood sugar control.*

# BAKED LEMON AND ALMOND CHEESECAKE

I have always thought that the texture of baked cheesecake is so much more interesting than the 'raw' version – I hope you agree. It certainly keeps well and is very moreish – so make enough for two even if you are on your own. | Serves 2

---

75g/3oz curd or cream cheese

1 egg

grated rind and juice of 2 lemons

15g/½ oz pale muscovado sugar

4 tbsp full fat milk

15g/½ oz flaked almonds

6 tbsp Greek yogurt

1 scant tsp honey

---

Heat the oven to 150C/300F/Gas mark 2.

In a bowl beat the cheese, egg, rind and juice of one of the lemons, the sugar and the milk.

Pour it into a small flan dish. Carefully sprinkle the almonds over the top and bake for 35 minutes. Remove and cool.

Meanwhile beat the remaining lemon rind and juice and the honey into the yogurt until they are well mixed.

Serve the cheesecake with the yogurt sauce.

> Lemon juice is good for diabetics as it boosts the levels of stomach acids which improves digestion and therefore the efficiency with which you digest carbohydrates.

# PEAR WITH CHOCOLATE AND GINGER WINE SAUCE

A very simple dish to make – yet it does look, and taste, delicious – and you can make it just for yourself. | Serves 1 (double quantities for 2)

---

1 slightly under-ripe pear

4 tbsp ginger wine

25g/1oz dairy-free dark chocolate – I use 85% cocoa solids but you may not wish to use quite such a bitter chocolate

2 tbsp cream, regular cow cream or soya or oat cream

---

Carefully peel the pear with a vegetable peeler and leave it whole. Sit it in the bottom of a small saucepan and pour round the wine. Cover the pan and simmer very gently for 15 minutes or until the pear is cooked – how long will depend on how under-ripe it is.

Meanwhile break the chocolate into small pieces into the cream and heat very slowly, stirring regularly, until the chocolate melts. Take off the heat.

When the pear is cooked transfer it to a serving dish and carefully stir the ginger wine into the chocolate sauce. Allow to cool but not get cold.

With a spoon, carefully pour/dribble some chocolate sauce over the pear so that it can drip down the sides and spoon the rest of the sauce into the bottom of the dish. Serve at room temperature.

> If you are concerned about your fat levels, especially your saturated fat levels, you may wish to substitute oat or soya cream for cow's milk cream. Both are really excellent (you can buy them in small long-life packs in most health food stores and many supermarkets).

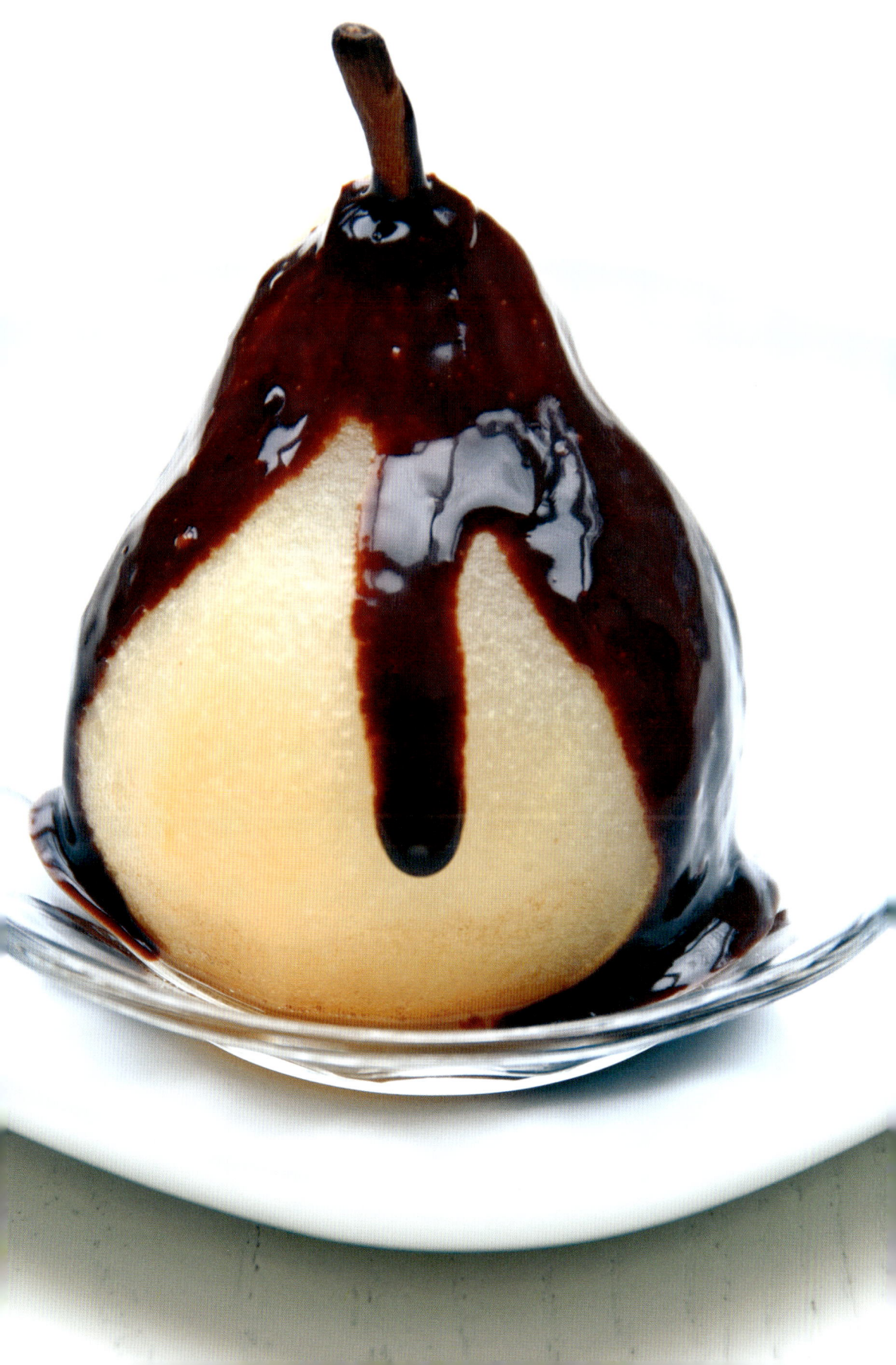

## CHOCOLATE POTS

This is such an easy recipe, but tastes so surprisingly good, that I keep coming back to it. Even if you are on your own, make enough for two as it will sit happily in the fridge for a couple of days so you will not feel as though you are 'eating it up'. | Serves 2

---

10g/scant ½ oz cornflour

150ml/¼ pint milk – cow, soya, oat or rice

25g/1oz dark, dairy-free chocolate

a couple of berries, a little icing sugar or some grated chocolate to decorate

---

In a pan mix the milk gradually into the cornflour until it is a smooth paste then heat slowly, stirring continually until it thickens.

Break the chocolate into the pan and stir until it melts.

Pour into 2 individual pots or ramekin dishes and chill.

Decorate with berries or a little extra grated chocolate to serve.

> Dark chocolate, the darker the better, is low on the Glycaemic Index as it has relatively little sugar – and a great chocolate hit! And if you find it too bitter on its own, the recipe above is a great way of taking the edge off it.

## CHOCOLATE STRAWBERRIES

This is an incredibly simple dessert – and can really give a lift to a meal on your own – or be fun if there are two of you as you can both coat your own strawberries – dipping them in the chocolate as if it were a fondue.

Pick strawberries that have good stems to hold on to while you are dipping.

---

3-6 strawberries per person

approx 50g/2oz dairy-free chocolate per person

---

Over a low heat, melt the chocolate in a small pan.

Set out a rack to receive the strawberries so that the chocolate can cool.

Holding the strawberries by the stem, dip them in the chocolate and cover the end, the side or as much of the strawberry as you fancy.

Stand on the rack and leave to cool and harden for 2-3 hours – or eat at once.

# BAKING

WHOLEMEAL BLUEBERRY MUFFINS
BANANA AND POLENTA BREAD
CINNAMON FLAPJACKS
OLD FASHIONED GINGER AND HONEY BISCUITS
LEMON SHORTBREADS
CHOCOLATE BROWNIES
CHOCOLATE AND PLUM CAKE
SERIOUSLY NUTTY CHRISTMAS OR FRUIT CAKE
RICH SEEDY CAKE
LEMON POPPY SEED CAKE

# WHOLEMEAL BLUEBERRY MUFFINS

Muffins are always good for that Sunday-morning-with-the-papers breakfast. If you want to keep some for next weekend, you can freeze two successfully. Allow them to thaw slowly at room temperature when you want to eat them – they won't take long. | Makes 3-4 smallish muffins

---

25g/1oz Demerara sugar
25g/1oz butter or coconut oil
1 small egg
4 tbsp fresh milk or buttermilk
70g/2½ oz wholemeal flour
1 scant tsp baking powder
small pinch of salt
40g/1½ oz blueberries

---

Heat the oven to 180C/350F/Gas mark 4.

Beat the sugar, butter or coconut oil, egg and milk together with an electric or hand beater.

Mix the flour with the baking powder and salt and gradually beat them into the liquid mixture.

Fold in the berries and spoon the dough into greased mince pie or tart pans. Bake the muffins for 20 minutes.

Remove them, cool slightly on a rack and serve warm or at room temperature.

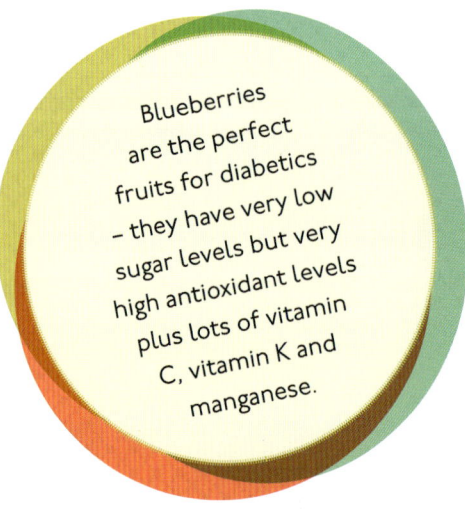

Blueberries are the perfect fruits for diabetics – they have very low sugar levels but very high antioxidant levels plus lots of vitamin C, vitamin K and manganese.

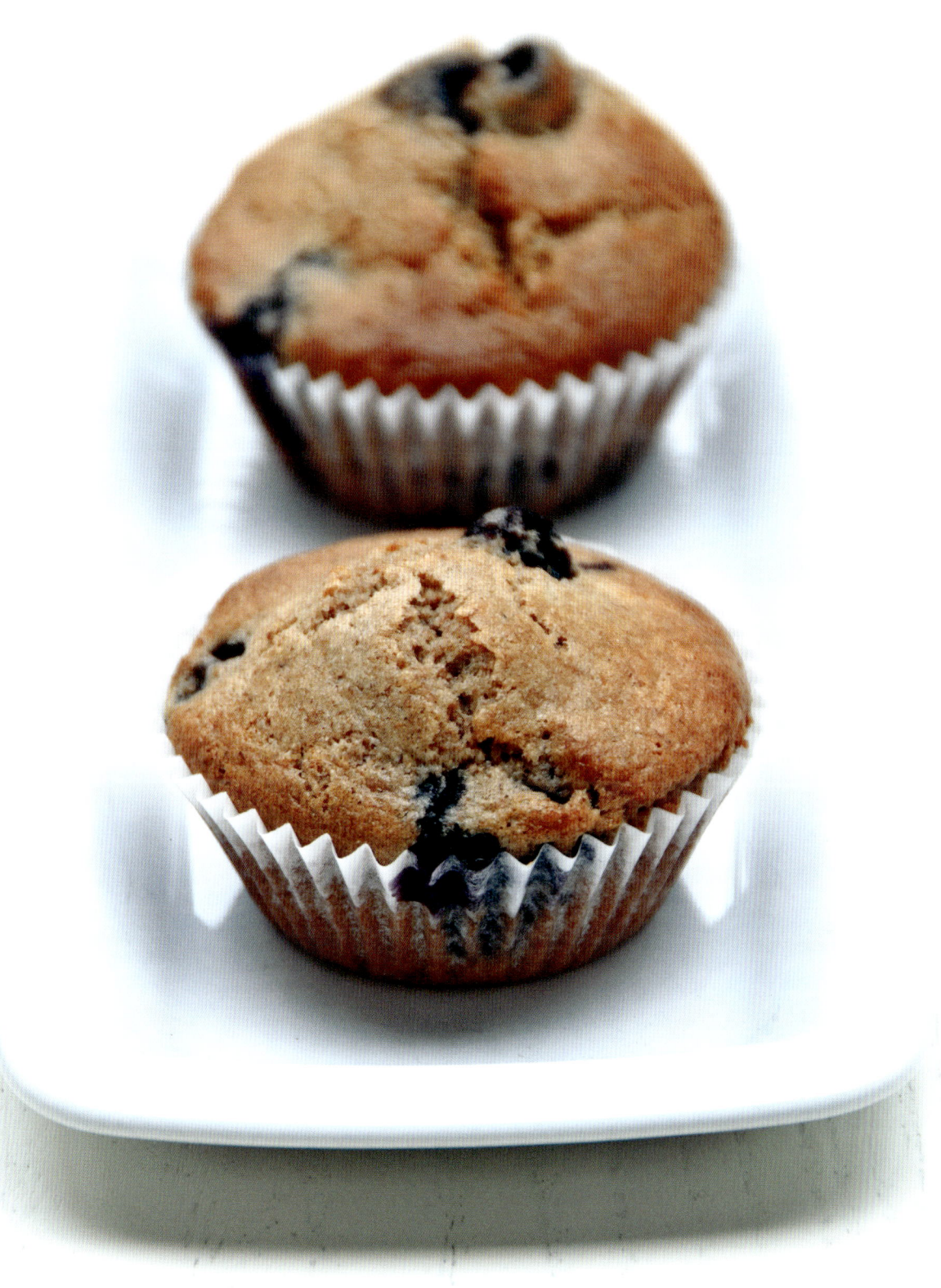

# BANANA AND POLENTA BREAD

This incredibly-easy-to-bake loaf makes one small loaf and freezes well so if you do not want to use the whole loaf, you do not need to. I do not add any sugar to the bread so it ends up as a cross between a bread and a cake – good both on its own or with butter. | Approx 10 slices

---

2 medium ripe bananas

175g/6oz coarse polenta

50g/2oz butter, spread or coconut oil

2 heaped tsp baking powder

pinch salt

1 egg

6 tbsp milk

---

Heat the oven to 180C/350F/Gas mark 4.

Purée the bananas in a food processor along with all the other ingredients. Line the base of a small loaf tin with greaseproof paper and oil its sides. Spoon the mixture into the tin and bake for 35 minutes or till a skewer comes out clean.

Remove from the oven and allow to cool slightly. Knock out of the tin and cool on a rack covered in a tea towel.

The Glycaemic Index/Load of bananas varies depending on how ripe they are because much of the carbohydrate in green or under-ripe bananas is in the form of a resistant starch which we cannot digest. As the banana ripens, the starch is converted into sugar. None the less, because of the large amount of fibre, even ripe bananas are OK for diabetics with an average on the Glycaemic Index of around 50.

# CINNAMON FLAPJACKS

Using sugar will give you a crunchier flapjack than if you use one of the liquid sweeteners – but both are delicious. You could also convert these into ginger flapjacks, if you prefer ginger, by substituting ground ginger for the cinnamon in the recipe. The seeds give a really interesting texture to the flapjacks. | Makes 4-6

---

50g/2oz butter, spread or coconut oil

1 tbsp agave syrup, maple syrup or honey or dark molasses sugar

50g/2oz porridge oats

1 level tbsp plain flour, wholemeal or white

scant 1 tsp of cinnamon (or ginger)

1 tbsp sunflower or pumpkin seeds

---

Heat the oven to 180C/350F/Gas mark 4.

Melt whichever fat you are using in a pan with the sweetener or sugar; stir over the heat for a minute or so. Add all the other ingredients and stir them thoroughly together – you should end up with a rather sticky mass.

Press it out into the bottom of a small baking tray or an ovenproof flan dish with your fingers – wooden spoons will just stick to it. It should be about 1 cm/½ inch (the thickness of your thumb) deep.

Cook the flapjacks for 18-20 minutes. Take them out of the oven, and with a knife, cut the mixture into wedges or fingers, depending on the shape of your dish. Leave them to cool a bit in the tin before carefully levering them out with a spatula or flexible knife and leaving them to cool completely on a wire rack before eating or storing.

Incidentally the crumbs which inevitably fall from the flapjacks are delicious sprinkled over yoghurt.

Agave syrup will, of course, give you the lowest Glycaemic Load in this recipe but remember that the fructose that it contains is not all good; honey and maple syrup are both rated as medium to low Glycaemic Load (they both also contain relatively high levels of fructose to glucose) but of course even dark molasses sugar is all glucose so high in terms of Glycaemic Load. However, it is being combined with very 'good' foods so you should not feel too bad if you wish to use it.

# OLD FASHIONED GINGER AND HONEY BISCUITS

The original of this recipe used black treacle but since honey has a far lower Glycaemic Load it might be well to substitute it. | Makes around 8 biscuits

---

100g/4oz sifted plain flour

scant ½ tsp ground ginger

40 g/1½ oz dark brown sugar

grated rind of 1 orange and 1 lemon

2 tbsp honey

40 g/1½ oz butter

---

Mix the flour, ginger, sugar and rind.

Melt the butter with the honey then add the dry ingredients. Mix to a stiff paste and chill for several hours or overnight. If you try to roll it out too soon it will be too soft to handle.

To bake, heat the oven to 180C/350F/Gas mark 4.

Roll out the mixture to approximately 5mm/¼inch thickness and stamp it out with a biscuit cutter or cut into shapes with a knife.

Bake in a hottish oven for 12-15 minutes taking care not to burn the biscuits. Cool on a rack.

*If you wanted to make gingerbread men, use a gingerbread man cutter (obtainable from any kitchen shop) then give him a face with two currants for eyes, a raisin for a nose and draw in his mouth with a knife point.*

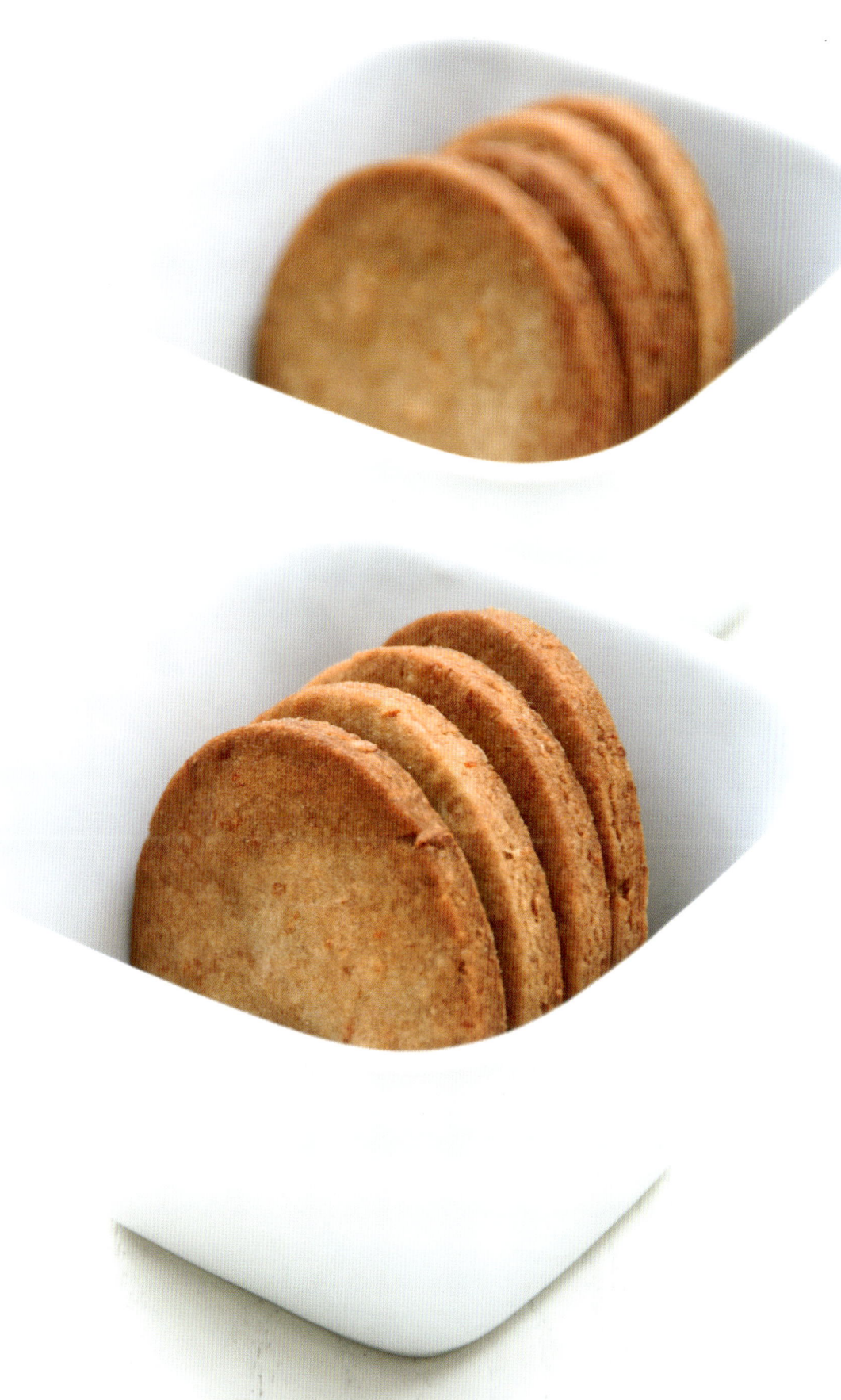

# LEMON SHORTBREADS

Lovely with a cup of coffee or tea.... | Makes approx 6 biscuits

---

25g/1oz butter or coconut oil
40g/1½oz pale muscovado sugar
grated rind of 1 small lemon
50g/2oz plain flour
25g/1oz ground almonds

---

Heat the oven to 160C/325F/Gas mark 3.

Beat the butter with the sugar and lemon rind with an electric or hand whisk until soft and light. Rub in the ground almonds and flour with your fingers, working as lightly as you can. Pat the mixture out into the bottom of a tin or shape it into a round approximately 20cm thick and bake for 15 minutes.

Remove and cut the break points (it should make around 6 biscuits) with a knife then return to the oven for another 5 minutes. Cool slightly then cut along the score marks and remove carefully, with a spatula, to a rack to get quite cold.

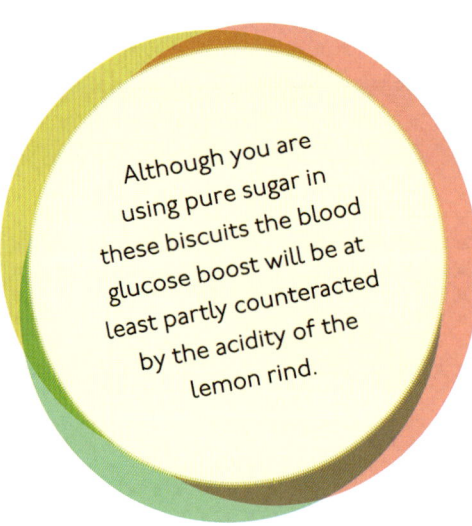

Although you are using pure sugar in these biscuits the blood glucose boost will be at least partly counteracted by the acidity of the lemon rind.

# CHOCOLATE BROWNIES

Makes 6 generous brownies or 8 smaller

150g/5oz low-fat spread
150g/5oz dark muscovado sugar
50g/2oz cocoa powder
50g/2oz porridge oats, whizzed in a processor to a coarse powder
50g/2oz sifted gram/chickpea flour
50g/2oz buckwheat flour
3 level tsp wheat and gluten free baking powder
150ml/¼ pint milk
50g/2oz broken walnuts

Preheat the oven to 160C/325F/Gas mark 3.

With an electric mixer beat the spread thoroughly with the sugar and the cocoa.

Fold in the flours and baking powder alternately with the milk, then fold in the walnuts.

Spoon the mixture into a well oiled square or rectangular tin, smooth out with a spatula and bake for 30 minutes or till a skewer comes out clean.

Cool for a few minutes in the tin then cut into whatever sized brownies you fancy.

Remove them carefully from the tin with a spatula and cool on a rack.

# CHOCOLATE AND PLUM CAKE

This is a lovely cake to make when fresh plums are around but, out of season, you could also use soft Agen prunes. If you are making it with the prunes, reduce the sugar to 75g/3oz as the prunes are that much sweeter than the fresh plums.

---

100g/4oz butter or low fat spread

100g/4oz dark muscovado sugar (75g/3oz if you are using prunes)

40g/1½oz cocoa powder

4 ripe fresh plums, stoned

2 medium eggs

50g/2oz wholemeal flour mixed with

50g/2oz fine porridge oats or rolled oats whizzed in a food processor

1 level tsp wheat and gluten free baking powder

40g/1½oz dark chocolate, nibbed

good quality plum jam (optional)

---

Heat the oven to 180C/350F/Gas mark 4.

Beat the butter or spread with the sugar with a hand or electric mixer until soft and creamy. Add the cocoa powder.

Purée three of the plums (or prunes) in a food processor or mash them by hand and add them to the mix. Add the eggs, one at a time, each with a spoonful of the flour and oat mix.

Chop the remaining plum (or prune) into fairly small pieces.

With a wooden spoon, fold in the remains of the flour, the baking powder, chocolate nibs and the plums (or prunes) into the mixture.

Grease a small (15cm/6 inch) loose-bottomed cake tin, or line it with greased greaseproof paper if it doesn't have a loose bottom. Spoon in the mixture and bake for 40 minutes or until a skewer comes out clean.

Cool for a few minutes in the tin then turn out onto a rack.

When cooled to room temperature, you can split the cake horizontally and fill with a good layer of plum jam if you want to – although that will increase the Glycaemic Load of the cake.

> If you are craving something sweet, a piece of cake which includes a whole load of nutrients as well as the sugar is a much better way to go than a KitKat bar.

# SERIOUSLY NUTTY CHRISTMAS OR FRUIT CAKE

Because of its high nut content and because it uses bananas as a sweetener rather than sugar, this is a really good cake for diabetics. Although bananas do have a strong flavour, there are so many other 'vigorous' ingredients in the cake that the bananas do not overpower. I suggest you make the full cake even if you are on your own as it keeps well, and if you really do have too much, you could halve, wrap it tightly and freeze it for an Easter treat.

---

100g/4oz butter, low fat spread or coconut oil

2 medium ripe bananas

rind and juice 2 lemons

2 large eggs, lightly beaten

75g/3oz each raisins and sultanas

150g/5oz soft dried apricots, chopped roughly

25g/1oz each flaked almonds and pine nuts

50g/2oz broken walnuts/pecans

50g/2oz toasted hazelnuts, chopped roughly

75g/3oz fine porridge oats or rolled oats, lightly pulverised in a food processor

75g/3oz plain flour

2 tsp baking powder

2 tsp ground nutmeg

1 tsp each ground ginger and ground cinnamon

2 tbsp brandy/orange/apple juice

---

Heat the oven to 160C/325F/Gas mark 3.

Purée the butter or spread with the banana and lemon rind and juice in a food processor.

Turn into a bowl and stir in the eggs followed by the fruits and nuts, followed by the flours, baking powder, spices and, finally, the brandy or fruit juice. Make sure that it is well mixed.

Line a 15cm/6 inch cake tin with greased greaseproof paper and spoon in the mixture. Smooth out and bake for 1 hour or till a skewer comes out clean. Cool slightly in the tin then turn out and leave to get completely cold before cutting as it can be quite crumbly.

*Apricots, of which there are lots in this cake, are one of the lowest dried fruits on the Glycaemic Index and have a very low Glycaemic Load – so you can feel free to have a second slice.*

# RICH SEEDY CAKE

This is a classic 'seedy cake' – a Madeira mixture with caraway seeds – perfect with a glass of Madeira! If you are not that keen on caraway seeds, and want just a plain Madeira cake, leave out the seeds and the spices. This makes a small cake which will keep you going for a few days – but if it is too much, halve it and freeze half. But make sure you wrap it well to freeze (otherwise it will dry out) and leave it to defrost slowly.

---

100g/4oz soft butter or low fat spread

75g/3oz light muscovado sugar

2 eggs, separated

1 scant tsp caraway seeds

½ level tsp each of ground nutmeg and cinnamon

100g/4oz plain flour

---

Heat the oven to 180C/350F/Gas mark 4.

Beat the butter with the sugar till it is light and fluffy in a mixer or with a hand whisk. Add the egg yolk with the caraway seeds and the spices and mix well.

Whisk the whites till they just hold their shape and fold them into the mixture along with the flour. Make sure they are well amalgamated. Spoon the mixture into a well greased, small loaf tin. If you are concerned about getting it out, line the tin with greased greaseproof paper.

Bake the cake for 40 minutes or till a skewer comes out clean. Remove it from the tin and allow it to cool on a rack before cutting.

*When this recipe was first written down in the mid 18th century, the roller mill had not yet been invented so 'fine white flour' would actually have been what we think of as a fine wholemeal flour. If you want to get the full 18th century feel, use wholemeal rather than white flour.*

# LEMON POPPY SEED CAKE

This cake is the base for the classic lemon drizzle cake but the drizzle icing is not great for diabetics as it is made from icing sugar although this is combined with helpful lemon juice. However, although on the whole I prefer not to use alternative sweeteners, this is a case where you might wish to use Xylitol in the cake itself so that you could then have your sugar allowance on the icing.

This amount makes a small loaf cake but if this is too much, it will freeze well for future use. However, if you are going to freeze it, do so before you ice it and ice the remaining half when it has been defrosted.

---

175g/6oz butter or low fat spread
175g/6oz caster sugar or light muscovado sugar or xylitol product such as Perfect Sweet
2 large eggs
175g/6oz self raising flour, sieved
1-2 lemons, depending on size
1 tbsp poppy seeds
2 gently heaped tbsp icing sugar

---

Heat the oven to 180C/350F/Gas mark 4.

Beat the butter or spread with the sugar in an electric mixer for 3-5 minutes or until it is light and fluffy.

Grate the rind from the lemon.

One at a time lightly beat in the eggs with a tablespoon of flour then fold in the rest of the flour along with the lemon rind, the poppy seeds and the juice of ½ a lemon.

Line a small loaf tin with oiled greaseproof paper.

Spoon the mixture into the tin and tap the cake tin gently a few times on the counter top to flatten out the top.

Bake for 45 minutes or until a skewer comes out clean. Remove from the oven, allow to cool for a few minutes and then remove from the tin onto a rack and allow to cool completely.

When the cake is cold, put the icing sugar in a small bowl and stir in up to 5 tsp of lemon juice – you want the icing to be quite thick but spreadable. Spoon it onto the top of the cake and then smooth it out with a spatula dipped in hot water, allowing the drips to run down the side of the cake.

Leave to dry before cutting.

> Xylitol is useful because not only does it have a very low Glycaemic Index but it is low in calories as well so good for weight control. You should be able to use it in the same quantities as you would sugar and although it does not deliver the same flavour as a muscovado sugar, it does mean that you can have a sweet cake without sending your blood sugars rocketing.

# INDEX

## A
agave syrup 141
Ajwar 28
Alcohol 15
Almond 119, 126
    almond, & lemon cheesecake 133
Alternative remedies 9
Anchovies 40, 62, 85, 90
Apple 56, 103, 129
    apple & berry crumble 124
    apple & cranberry clafoutis 128
    apple, & chicken salad 94
Apricots 147
Artichoke hearts 95
Aubergine 28
Avocado, spinach & mozzarella salad 107

## B
Baked lemon & almond cheesecake 133
Balsamic vinegar 96
Banana & polenta bread 140
Bean, & sausage pot 84
Beef
    casserole 66
    bobotie 67
    minced with curly kale 69
    pot roast 64
    steak with garlic 70
Beet leaves 103

Beetroot
    & chickpea salad 100
    & red cabbage with rollmops 51
    with sausages 88
Berry & apple crumble 124
Biscuits, ginger & honey 142
Blood sugar control 10, 11
Blueberry muffins 138
Bobotie 67
Bread, banana & polenta 140
Broad beans 34
Broccoli, and pasta au gratin 44
Brownies, chocolate 145
Brussels sprout & celeriac salad 104
Bulgar wheat 108
Butter beans 88
Butter bean & beetroot salad 100
Butternut squash ratatouille 106

## C
Cabbage
    red casserole 114
    red with beetroot 51
    with gammon 86
Cakes
    chocolate & plum 146
Christmas 147
Christmas upside down 129
    fruit 147
    lemon & poppy seed 149
    rich seedy 148
Capers 40
Carrot & red lentil soup 18

Cashew nut & cauliflower salad 102
Casserole, red cabbage 114
Cauliflower 90
  && cashew nut salad 102
  au gratin 44
Cavolo nero with beet leaves 103
Celeriac 117
  & Brussels sprout salad 104
  soup 20
  with kale & pecan nuts 111
Cheese
  blue 44
  mozzarella 107
Cheesecake, baked lemon & almond 133
Chestnuts 116
  with lamb's kidneys 76
  with pheasant 118
Chicken
  & apple salad 94
  breasts with orange & artichoke hearts 95
  salad with pumpkin oil 96
  soup 92
  with anchovy & cauliflower 90
  with okra 91
  oven-baked 92
Chickpea & beetroot salad 100
Chilli with cod 60
Chillies 50
Chinese medicine 9
Chocolate
  & ginger wine sauce 134
  & plum cake 146
  brownies 145
  pots 136
  strawberries 136
Chorizo 120
Christmas cake 147
Christmas upside down cake 129
Cinnamon flapjacks 141
Clafoutis, apple & cranberry 128
Coconut milk crème 126
Coconut oil 132
Cod with chilli 60
Coriander 110
Crab, ginger & almond soufflé 119
Cracked wheat with spinach & pine nuts 108
Cranberry & apple clafoutis 128
Crumble
  Apple & berry 124
  Oaty strawberry 132

## D

Diabetes mellitus 8
Dried fruits 130
Duck with ginger & water chestnuts 98

## E

Egg & lentil pie 33
Eggs
  au miroir 36
  Hard boiled with spinach 38
  Herb frittata 34
  Spinach soufflé 32

## F

Faisant aux chataignes 118
Fennel
  & strawberry salad 112
  & leek soup 21
  with salmon 54
Fettucine with smoked salmon 42

Fish
  Cod with chilli 60
  Haddock, smoked chowder 22
  Haddock, smoked pie 58
  Herrings, rollmops 51
  Mackerel baked with apple 56
  Mackerel, smoked 20
  Mackerel, smoked with curly kale 55
  Salmon in Parma ham 122
  Salmon with fennel & tomatoes 54
  Poached trout with rhubarb sauce 59
  Smoked haddock chowder 22
  Smoked haddock pie 58
  Smoked salmon, with fettucine 42
  Tuna with mangetout 57
Flapjacks, cinnamon 141
Frittata 34
Fructose 16
Fruit cake 147
Fruit salad, hot 130
Fruits, dried 130
Fusilli with capers & anchovies 40

# G

Gammon with green lentils & cabbage 86
Ginger 48, 66, 92, 98, 119
   & honey biscuits 142
Ginger wine & chocolate sauce 134
Gingerbread men 142
Glycaemic index 13
Glycaemic load 13
Good foods 14

# H

Haddock, smoked chowder 22
Haddock, smoked pie 58

Ham 120
Harissa 75
Herb frittata 34
Herrings, rollmops 51
Honey & ginger biscuits 142
Horseradish 88, 104
Hot fruit salad 130
Hot plum dessert 125
Hyperglycaemia 11, 12
Hypoglycaemia 11, 12

# J

Jambalaya 120

# K

Kale 69
   and warm pasta salad 43
   curly with smoked mackerel 55
   with celeriac & pecan nuts 111
Kebabs, lamb & pepper 79
Kidney soup 23
Kidneys, lamb with chestnuts & marsala 76

# L

Lamb
   & pepper kebabs 79
   shoulder, oyster stuffed 78
   Tajine 74
   Rack of with mustard crust 80
   Kidneys with chestnuts & marsala 76
Leek & fennel soup 21
Lemon poppy seed cake 149
Lemon shortbreads 144
Lemon, baked cheesecake 133
Lentil(s)
   & egg pie 33

green with gammon 86
red soup 18
with okra & coriander 110
Limes 48

## M

Mackerel baked with apple 56
Mackerel, smoked 20
Mackerel, smoked with curly kale 55
Mangetout 57
Marinade 79
Marsala 76
Miso 21
Moules marinières 52
Mozzarella, spinach & avocado salad 107
Muffins, wholemeal blueberry 138
Mushroom soup, cream of 30
Mussels 52
Mustard crust 80

## N

New Orleans jambalaya 120
Nutritional therapy 11
Nuts 147

## O

Oat cream 42, 59, 134
Oaty raspberry crumble 132
Oaty strawberry crumble 132
Offal 23
Oil, coconut 132
Okra
 & salami savoury 26
 with chicken 91
 with lentils & coriander 110
Orange 95

Oven-baked chicken with ginger 92
Oxtail stew 68
Oyster stuffed lamb shoulder 78

## P

Parma ham 122
Pasta
 and broccoli au gratin 44
 Fettucine with smoked salmon 42
 Fusilli with capers & anchovies 40
 Spaghetti carbonara 46
 Warm salad with curly kale 43
Pear
 with chocolate & ginger wine sauce 134
Pepper & anchovy salad 62
Pecan nuts 111
Pepper, and lamb kebabs 79
Pepper, pear & anchovy salad 62
Pheasant with chestnuts 118
Pie
 Lentil & egg 33
 Smoked haddock 58
Pigeon breasts with chestnuts 116
Pine nuts 108
Pita 75, 79
Plum
 & chocolate cake 146
 Hot dessert 125
Poached trout with rhubarb sauce 59
Polenta & banana bread 140
Poppy seed & lemon cake 149
Pork chops with apple & rosemary 85
Port 121
Potatoes, baked 56
Prawns 120
 stir fried with ginger 48

Prunes 116
Pumpkin oil, with chicken 96

## R
Rack of lamb with mustard crust 80
Raspberry crumble 132
Ratatouille with butternut squash 106
Red cabbage casserole 114
Red pepper 28
Redcurrants 121
Rhubarb sauce 59
Rice 57, 67
Rich seedy cake 148
Rosemary 85

## S
Salad
  Beetroot & chickpea 100
  Brussels sprout & celeriac 104
  Butter bean & beetroot 100
  Cauliflower & cashew nut 102
  Cavolo nero with beet leaves 103
  Celeriac with kale & pecan nuts 111
  Chicken & apple 94
  Chicken with pumpkin oil 96
  Cracked wheat with spinach & pine nuts 108
  Fennel & strawberry 112
  Hot fruit 130
  Lentils with okra & coriander 110
  Pepper, pear & anchovy 62
  Seafood 50
  Spinach, avocado & mozzarella 107
  Warm pasta and curly kale 43
Salami & okra savoury 26
Salmon in Parma ham 122
Salmon with fennel & tomatoes 54

Sauce
  Chocolate & ginger wine 134
  Rhubarb 59
Sausage & bean pot 84
Sausages with beetroot 88
Seafood salad 50
Seaweeds 22, 55
Seeds 43
Seedy cake 148
Shortbreads, lemon 144
Slow cook pot roast 64
Smoked haddock chowder 22
Smoked haddock pie 58
Smoked salmon, with fettucine 42
Soufflé, crab, ginger & almond 119
Soufflé, spinach 32
Soup
  Carrot & red lentil 18
  Celeriac 20
  Chicken 92
  Cream of mushroom 30
  Kidney 23
  Leek & fennel 21
  Smoked haddock chowder 22
  Watercress 24
Soya cream 42, 59, 134
Spaghetti carbonara 46
Spinach
  Avocado & mozzarella salad 107
  Soufflé 32
  with cracked wheat & pine nuts 108
  with hard boiled eggs 38
Squash, butternut 66
Squash, butternut ratatouille 106
Steak with garlic 70
Steaming 54
Stew
  Jambalaya 120

Oxtail 68
Stir fried prawns with ginger 48
Tuna with mangetout 57
Strawberries
   Chocolate 136
   & fennel salad 112
   crumble 132
Sweeteners 15

## T

Tagine, lamb 74
Tomatoes, with salmon 54
Trout, poached 59
Tuna stir fried with mangetout 57
Turkey breast with orange & artichoke hearts 95

## V

Venison braised with port 121

## W

Warm pasta and curly kale salad 43
Water chestnuts 98
Watercress soup 24
Wheat
   bulgar 108
   cracked with spinach & pine nuts 108
Wholemeal blueberry muffins 138

## X

Xylitol 149

## Y

Yellow split peas 92

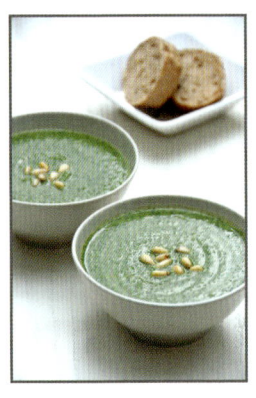
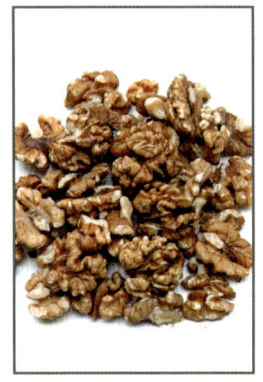
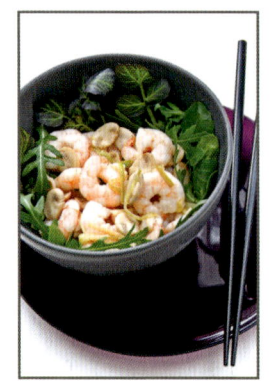
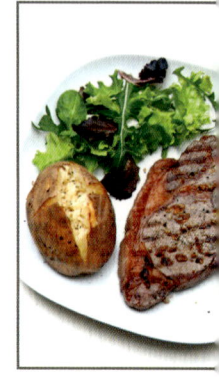
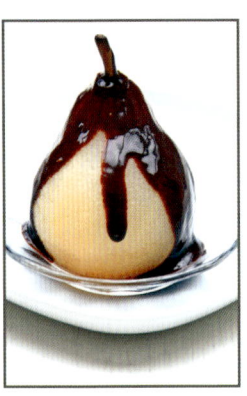
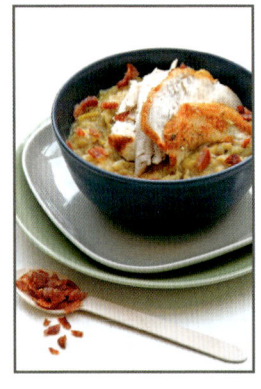
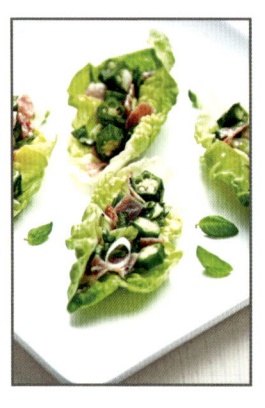
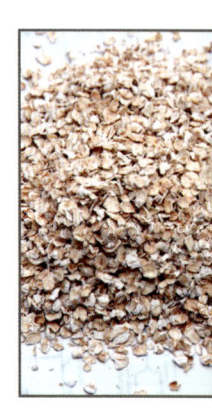
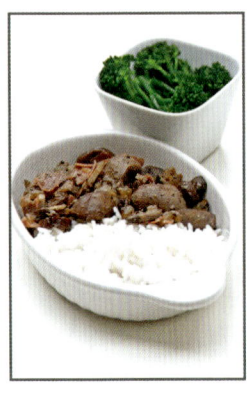
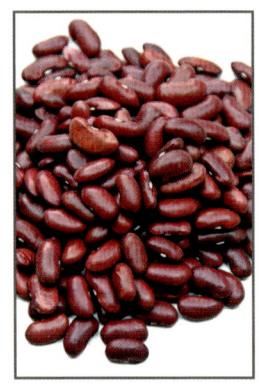
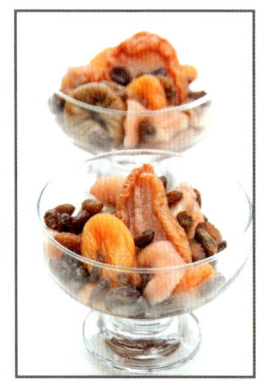
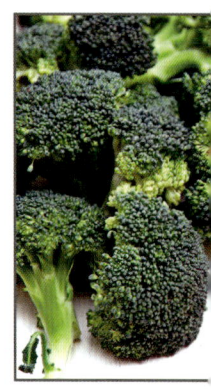
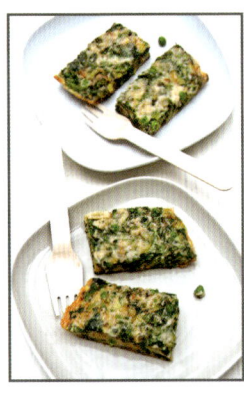
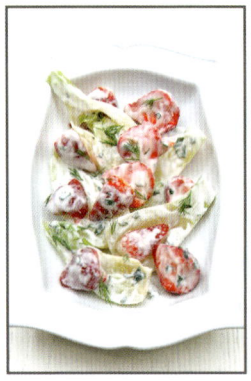
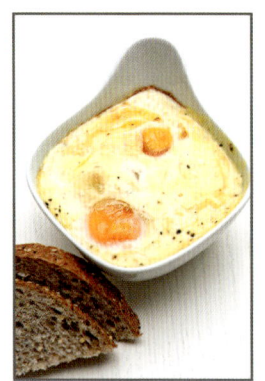
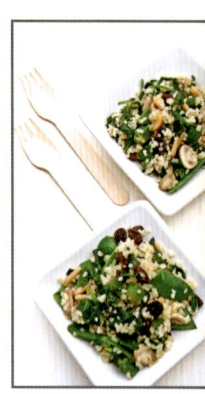

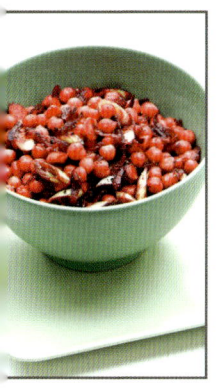
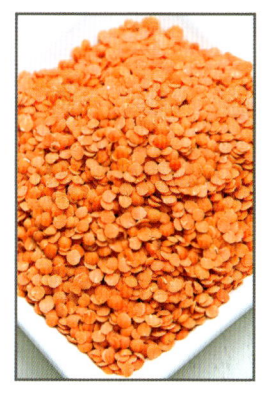
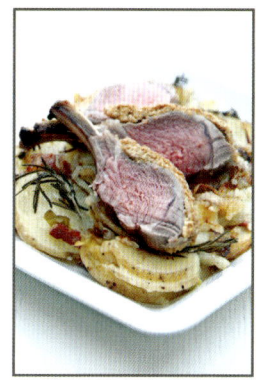
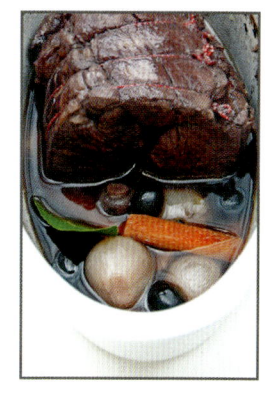
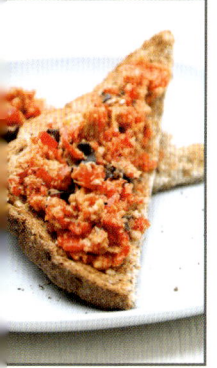
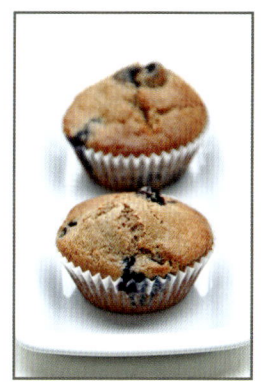
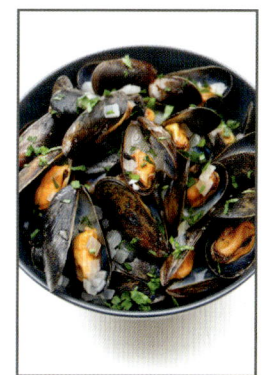
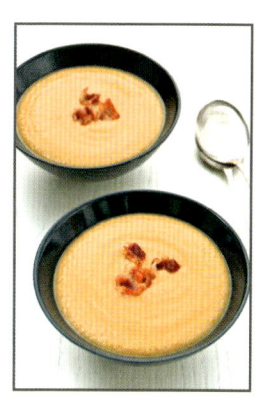
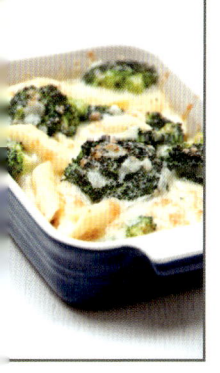
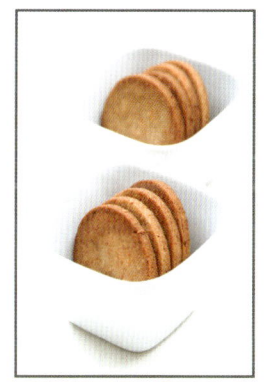
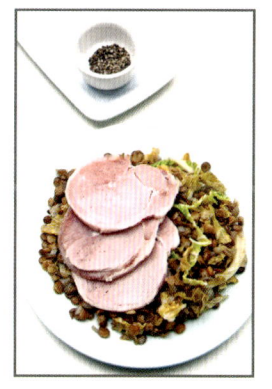
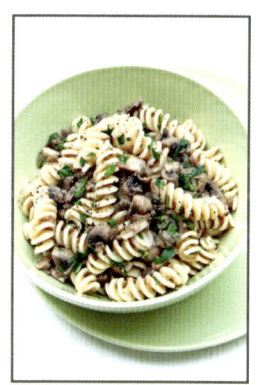
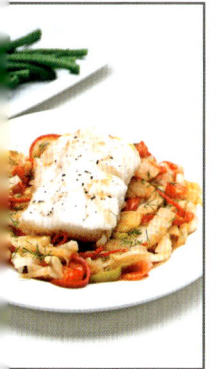
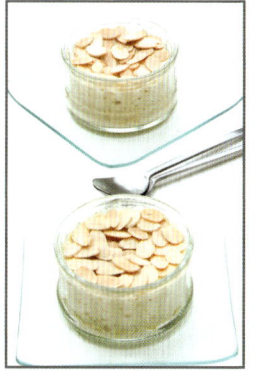
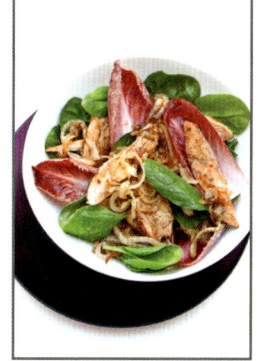
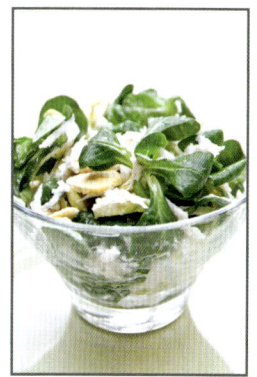

AT-A-GLANCE GALLERY

# ALSO BY
# MICHELLE BERRIEDALE-JOHNSON

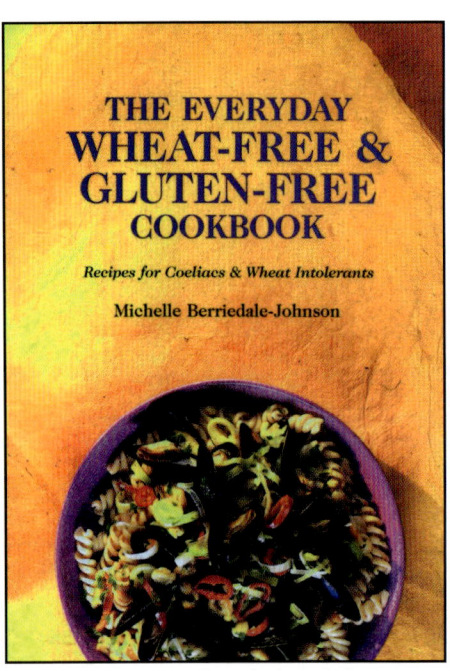

## THE EVERYDAY WHEAT-FREE & GLUTEN-FREE COOKBOOK

### Recipes for Coeliacs & Wheat Intolerants

- 224 pages •
- 248 x 175mm •
- 12pp of colour •
- paperback •
- £10.99 •
- ISBN 978-1-898697-90-9 •

If you suffer from gluten allergy or intolerance (Coeliac disease), or wheat intolerance, then you probably know the only treatment for either of these debilitating conditions is a gluten-free and wheat-free diet – this means eliminating bread, biscuits, crispbreads, cakes, pastry, pasta, breadcrumbs, semolina and food cooked in batter, as well as many tinned, packaged and processed foods – in fact foods which usually form the greater part of a normal day-to-day diet.

Michelle Berriedale-Johnson, a leading expert and author in the field of food allergies and nutrition, has developed this original collection of recipes using both wheat flour alternatives as well as the gluten-free flours, breads and pastas now available.

If you're worried about what to eat and how to eat, and you're stuck for recipes for balanced meals, then this book is for you.

- Over 200 specially created wheat-free and gluten-free recipes •
- Proprietary gluten-free flours, bread and cake mixes tried, tested and recommended •
- The very latest medical and dietary findings •
- Nutritional analysis for each recipe •